Leaving This Life with Hospice

Stories of Wonder and Hope

Margaret Ledger

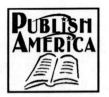

PublishAmerica
Baltimore

First printing

ISBN: 1-4137-7998-0
PUBLISHED BY PUBLISHAMERICA, LLLP
www.publishamerica.com
Baltimore

Printed in the United States of America

Acknowledgments

I started writing this story ten years ago, when, as a new hospice volunteer, I called my manager to tell her a story of one of my first hospice patients. She asked me to put the story in writing because she thought other people would like to read it. That was the beginning.

My son, Aron, and my daughter, Deena, have encouraged me to write for years, and continued to do so throughout this process. My husband, Peter, always offers me encouragement on the things I feel passionate about. I thank him, too, for ignoring my complaints.

Many friends read early collections of stories. Their feedback on the need for clarification and explanation made me realize that I needed to write a book. Eight people read my first draft and encouraged me to push on. Most publishers didn't want to hear from a first-time writer with such a title. That was when Peter suggested I make 10 copies and give them away. So I did. Then one reader, Roger Brandt, liked it, and asked whether I would like him to tell his sister about it. "By the way," he said, "did I tell you she's a literary agent?"

So that is how I was introduced to Nan DeBrandt. Without her encouragement and personal persistence, this book would never have seen the light of day.

Many more friends read various revisions and gave me feedback and edits. Moya Daly edited a major portion of the text for me. I was also delighted to get support and a forward from Ira Byock, M.D. Working with PublishAmerica has been a very positive experience.

To all these people, named and unnamed, I am truly grateful. Most of all, I thank the patients and families, who were willing for me to share their special stories. I am also grateful to the hospice organization itself, and to the wonderful hospice employees and volunteers, who are truly dedicated to making a difference in the world, one person at a time. I am honored to work with them.

Contents

Foreword

Dying is the last thing on most people's minds. More accurately, it's in a back corner of our minds. We keep it there, as if in a dark closet. As we age and experience the death of others, the fact that life eventually, inevitably, ends constantly rattles the closet door. When serious illness or injury strikes ourselves or someone we love, considerable energy is required to suppress thoughts of dying and death. Denial can be exhausting as mortal thoughts constantly threaten to erupt into conscious awareness. Dying is inherently hard, but our unrelenting efforts to deny, ignore or avoid the inevitable makes it much harder.

Misconceptions about dying and death abound. People's beliefs are based on variable amounts of personal experience and lots of media portrayals. Unfortunately, misinformation often carries grave consequences. Most people presume that dying and suffering are intertwined. We turn away, hoping that when death does come, it will be painless and quick.

Compounding matters, our culture tends to conflate dying with death, psychologically and linguistically. It's common to read or hear the word "death" used when, although grammatically permissible, the word "dying" would have been a better fit. Death is a lifeless state that occurs after a person dies. In contrast, dying is a part of living. If we ignore the distinction between dying and death we may assume that a terminally ill person's life is already over. As the stories in *Leaving This Life with Hospice* reveal, nothing could be further from the truth.

Whether in agony or bliss or, for most, somewhere in between, people often live intensely during the time we label "dying."

For those of us who seek to be of help to people who are dying, Yogi Berra's wise admonition applies: "It ain't over 'til it's over." It's not unusual to hear a seriously ill person referred to in the past tense. ("I'm sorry to hear that Mrs. Jenkins is so ill. She was such a nice lady.") Assuming that a person's life is over before it's over can lead to nihilism. If we presume to already know the end of a person's story, why bother trying to change it? I have the same concern about the old saw, "People die as they have lived." At best, it is a dangerous half-truth. Of course, some people live through their last breath in the identical manner in which they have through their life. But it is also true that during their last months many people change, in personal and interpersonal ways, and that they often do so quite deliberately.

Every human being remains unique through the moment of death. Still, clinicians in hospice and palliative care recognize important commonalities of human experience as people deal with issues of completion and life closure. When people do not die as they have lived, the changes are almost always in becoming more reflective, introspective, emotionally honest and vulnerable.

It's common for people to reach out to others whom they love, at times across great geographic and emotional gulfs.

When important relationships have been fractured in the past, people may seize the final chance to make amends. I've seen more than a few angry, gruff, suspicious people gradually soften, and open up emotionally to their families and others. One man who fits this profile who was living with advanced lung cancer told me, "I have grown more in the last year than I did my whole adult life."

As difficult as dying is, acknowledging that time is limited can be a remarkable stimulus for growth. It offers a chance to reflect on what would be left undone and unsaid if one were to die today. It provides the opportunity, if a person so chooses, to ask for and offer forgiveness, to express appreciation and love.

People who are dying may be drawn inward to explore questions relating to their place in the world, the meaning of their individual life and life in general. Even those who have never been metaphysically inclined, may find themselves earnestly wondering what awaits them after death. As Ledger's personal experiences and stories illustrate, in drawing close to death many people enter a realm in which the past and present intertwine and death is separated from life by the sheerest of films. The tendency is to consider such experiences as a type of delirium risks dismissing the unexplainable with a diagnosis. Better to admit we don't know. Phenomena such as prescient dreams and the uncanny sense of the presence of their deceased loved ones that bereaved people frequently describe challenge us to admit that our world is more mysterious than we understand.

Although we are culturally conditioned to expect suffering, positive personal experiences at the end of life are not figments of poets', novelists' or hospice nurses' imagination. I'm no longer surprised when I hear a dying person say that they are happier or more at peace than they have ever been. Typically, however, it takes conscious work and considerable preparation for a person to die well. This is increasingly true in the stressed, fragmented, treat-at-all-costs environment of contemporary health care. The hardest work, of course, falls to the person who is dying and his or her closest friends and family. However, we can help one another through this time and process. Each of us has a role to play, whether we are clinical professionals, a close friend or relative of a person who is dying, or merely a member of the person's extended community. How can we help? Most importantly, by showing up—even when it's inconvenient and you don't know what you can do. Most reliably, we can help by listening—even when the person we're listening to is feeling helpless and hopeless and we don't know what to say. Our time and attention are the most simple and profound gifts of service we can give.

A team of caring professionals, complemented by community volunteers, can make a world of difference. As a physician specializing in palliative care, my first priority clinically is to help people to be as comfortable as possible, ensuring that their attention is not trapped by constant pain or other distress. In addition to effectively treating symptoms, the caring team can help with myriad practical challenges of living with illness, caregiving at home and navigating the complexities of the health care system.

Recent advances in clinical sciences and in developing models of health service delivery of palliative care carry bright potential for improving the quality of life's end for millions in the future. Unfortunately, at present not everyone receives the sort of comprehensive care, skillful guidance and emotional support that is possible. Today, people who are ill and their families need knowledgeable and assertive advocates to ensure that they get the best care possible. Socially, culturally and politically we must continue striving to preserve the opportunity to die well.

While death will remain a mystery, always beyond our reach, dying is the most universal and natural of human experiences. The stories that fill *Leaving This Life with Hospice* provide reassurance that we will all get through this final transition. In simple fact, despite all our struggles to cling to life, the vast majority of people leave this life gently with at least a brief preceding sense of well-being. As Margaret Ledger reveals, this is part of the final mystery, too.

Ira Byock, M.D.
Director of Palliative Care, Dartmouth-Hitchcock Medical Center.
Author of *Dying Well* and *The Four Things That Matter Most.*

Introduction

Few of us, especially by mid-life, have been left untouched by stories of death and dying. These experiences are unique and intensely personal. Some people are happy to recount their tale to anyone willing to listen, whereas others choose not to mention their grief ever again. I have found these people in the former category, listened to them and felt moved profoundly by the contents of all their narratives. They are quintessentially human revelations, each filled with hope, love and joy. I want to share them with you and trust that you will find something in them that speaks to you.

My first experience with terminally ill patients was as an assistant physicist in a radiotherapy ward in England. I was a recent physics graduate. My job was to monitor radiation equipment and to plan how the machines would deliver the dose of radiation that the doctor had prescribed, to the patients' tumors. I had to meet with patients and I talked at length with many of them. During this time I became quite upset about how we were trying to cure some terminally ill patients who would have preferred to be supported by the medical profession in dying peacefully. I knew I had no way of influencing the then medical profession to change their thinking, consequently I was glad to move away from that job and I forgot about those experiences for years.

At the age of fifty, I decided to offer myself as a hospice volunteer. I volunteered to work in a local hospice and did so for five years while still working elsewhere full time. I became the hospice bereavement coordinator, and subsequently I also became the volunteer coordinator. So my experiences with the dying and with the bereaved have evolved principally from the people I have been privileged to meet during my ten years of service with hospice.

When Death Comes

When death comes
like the hungry bear in autumn;
when death comes and takes all the bright coins from his purse

to buy me, and snaps the purse shut;
when death comes
like the measle-pox;

when death comes
like an iceberg between the shoulder blades,

I want to step through the door full of curiosity, wondering:
what is it going to be like, that cottage of darkness?

And therefore I look upon everything
as a brotherhood and a sisterhood,
and I look upon time as no more than an idea,
and I consider eternity as another possibility,

and I think of each life as a flower, as common
as a field daisy, and as singular,

and each name a comfortable music in the mouth,
tending, as all music does, toward silence,

and each body a lion of courage, and something
precious to the earth.

When it's over, I want to say: all my life
I was a bride married to amazement.
I was the bridegroom, taking the world in my arms.
When it's over, I don't want to wonder
if I have made of my life something particular, and real.
I don't want to find myself sighing and frightened,
or full of argument.

I don't want to end up simply visiting this world.

—from *New and Selected Poems* by Mary Oliver [*1]

Illness and Fear

I would like to beg you...to have patience with everything unresolved in your heart and try to love the questions themselves as if they were locked rooms or books written in a foreign language. Don't search for the answers, which could not be given to you now because you would not be able to live them and the point is to live everything. Live the questions now.
—From *LETTERS TO A YOUNG POET,* by Rainier Maria Wilke *²

If something is wrong with our bodies, our own fears can propel us quickly into our assumed conclusion. A lump! It must be cancer. We are promised a test, we wait for the test, and for the results, and in most cases fearing what might be said when the long wait for the results culminates. Our minds are subject to a plethora of fears until the results of the tests are received. Often our fears turn out to be totally misplaced, not to mention false. The reality of the diagnosis can be something commonplace and curable. However, one day, unless we die very suddenly, we will face a diagnosis of a potentially life-threatening illness.

Physicians are committed to saving and prolonging life; the

majority has had little or no training in caring for the dying. Modern medicine, both surgery and medication, can do wonders, so patients try one new drug or treatment after another. Treatment of cancer today has meant that patients can live longer and still be trying to effect a total cure right up to within a few hours of death. It is very difficult to know when to say "no" to more treatments and turn the focus to of the sick toward enjoying a good quality of life for the time, which remains until death.

Patients, families and friends are going to go through a whole range of tough emotions as the process of dying is going on. The patients might experience the following:

Denial: I am fine. I don't believe this is happening to me.
Anger: Why me? This isn't fair! This doctor is incompetent!
Guilt: Leaving my family who can't care for themselves.
Overwhelming sadness: Leaving everything I love?
Fear: What path will this illness take? Will I be alone? Will I be in pain? Dying is said to be the final stage of growth, and is likely to be the toughest. [*3]

No wonder this is a topic we don't think about. It arouses fear. Fear of the unknown is always lessened by information on what this experience has been like for others. If we can explore our fears and get answers to our questions, the fears will abate. Many people do die a peaceful death without fear in the later stages of their illness, though their malady may have been very hard. The path patients might have to travel to come to acceptance of the fact that they are dying might have been very difficult, but the final stage is often quiet and peaceful.

When the focus is on trying to achieve a cure, patients will undergo any therapy possible, and many of those attempts to cure are an extreme ordeal for everyone concerned. The patient cannot go through the steps of coming to closure on life while going through this day-to-day struggle with survival.

Fear

Nobody will ever pretend illness and death is anything but very difficult, but fear is the real crippler. Fear of pain and fear of being a burden are huge issues. Within these issues are encompassed fear of death, fear of no longer existing, fear of leaving loved ones who are ill-prepared to cope with life without their loved ones or life partners, and even fear of not being remembered. People don't seem to be able to embrace peace until they have looked at all their fears and have come to accept what is happening.

People seem to react differently with different diagnoses. The very word "cancer" is a total shock because people associate it with a death sentence: "The big C." If the disease is diagnosed as life threatening, patients and their families must come face to face with all their fears about loss. Chronic diseases such as emphysema or heart disease may also be life threatening, but often people fear living a greatly restricted life for a long time and being a burden to others. When I had back problems for years and lived with pain, I, too, feared becoming incapacitated and bed-ridden.

A nurse who worked with young patients with AIDS said her patients described their biggest fear as not being remembered. Remembrance work, such as the AIDS quilt or a commemorative wall at a local AIDS home, has helped many dying patients see that their name will live on.

Fear of pain is a very common fear. Control of pain and assistance in care, from hospice-like care, can make an enormous difference to a patient and their families. Those dying must be given information and support to make decisions about their own treatment. They should be given the dignity of choosing which strategy seems right to them. People tend to live the last stages of their life just the way they have always lived their lives. For example, occasionally people, who have always had to struggle in this life, may choose not to take sufficient medication to alleviate all pain. If they want to continue their struggle in their own way, then that should be their prerogative.

Knowledge and understanding also go a long way to relieve fear. If patients and their loved ones understand what is likely to happen and how they will be able to cope within the scope of their situation to maximum advantage of everybody at various times and stages, much of their fear can be alleviated.

Accepting a terminal diagnosis

Modern medicine can work wonders and cures us from many ills. Some people pull back time and time again, they cling to life when we believe they are close to the final stages of leaving it. Unwilling to face the reality that they or their loved one is dying, patient and relatives demand a system of most aggressive treatment to the end. Doctors are trained to cure and will continue to try anything in their power to do so, if that appears to be what the patients and families seek. In a culture that is ready to sue if the opportunity presents itself, modern hospitals continue to exhaust every medical option. Technology has advanced relentlessly and is continuing to do so, and therefore it becomes harder and harder to know when to accept that any disease is going to be terminal.

The greatest difficulty for those who are dying is that of acquiring a good understanding of the chances of overcoming a particular illness and the prices to be paid in the level of their body's ability to cope with the treatment. Sometimes the remedy so called can be as painful as the illness. Age is another key factor. Older people are going to have a harder time coping with treatments and their side effects. Sometime the question is how much more time of living is the treatment likely to provide and what is the physical cost? It is all a matter of probabilities. The doctors can give typical ranges of time. They are basing their judgments on the knowledge they have of previous patients' histories. Nevertheless, each patient is unique, mentally, physically and emotionally.

Relationships with the doctors are the keystone. If patients can ask questions and get comprehensive, honest answers at each stage it certainly helps. Doctors should be able to outline the possibilities; if we do this we have a 50/50 chance of success. If we do that we have a 10% chance of it helping. The patient needs to know the probabilities and the range of possible outcomes. They need to know, and more importantly understand, how they will be affected by each treatment. This means the patients should be informed regarding all the positive benefits and all the possible disadvantages of each avenue of possible treatment. Only then may they make a truly informed choice.

Patients need to let the doctors know how they want to balance treatment and hope of cure against comfort measures. They need to be able to tell the doctor how they rate life: is every possible minute of being alive important? Or would they prefer a shorter time with a higher probability of being made comfortable throughout the illness? One hopes that patients have doctors who will be open and honest, give the patients and their families the fullest account of all the information available and let them decide when to let go of the hope of cure and focus on the quality of time left, which can be lived in maximum comfort.

A work, which may facilitate a discussion, is the "Five Wishes Document."*[4] It helps patients and their families focus on the right questions to ask. The patient's decisions about treatment directions may well change as the disease progresses. Not only do the patients need to talk openly about their thoughts, feelings and beliefs with their doctors, but also with his family and friends. Close family of the afflicted needs to do the same, so that they can share fears of the process of their dying loved one or of life after the death.

Who makes the choices?

The patient should be the one to make the decisions on their treatment. We cannot expect all family members to come to the same conclusion simultaneously, but talking through how everyone else feels, helps them come to terms with both current and changing situations. Continuous communication is important, because the patient might change their outlook as the disease progresses; however, it is important that the patients feel they have some control as they make decisions.

I meet many people with serious regrets on this issue of choice after the death has occurred. Hindsight is wonderful, and it is helpful to acknowledge feelings of guilt and perhaps visualize what they would have done differently with the knowledge they now possess. I can always get them to acknowledge they did the very best they knew how at the time. After her husband's death, one woman shared tearfully, "I talked him into getting that treatment for me, because I couldn't bear to see him die. He knew he was dying, and he didn't want to go through that treatment again." I could only reassure her that she did the best she could at the time, given her own feelings and the information she was given.

Summary

Illness arouses all our fears. Fear can easily be exacerbated. With a chronic illness, or with recurring bouts of an acute problem, death may be years away. On the other hand death may be a very sudden reality. The crux of the matter seems to be how much living we put into the time that is left, once we know we are terminally ill.

I can only stand in awe of the people I have met who faced the reality of their approaching death with courage and love, made good their relationships, experienced love, and let go. Surviving family and friends have had incredible experiences during the illness of a relative, feeling hitherto unknown emotions, which have covered the gamut of their whole being intensely. Not least amongst these, the pain of their loss, the intensity of their love, both endured and enduring. Finally they are left knowing that the passing was as good as it could have been.

The Changing Environment of Medical Care

Care of the dying

Once upon a time, death was viewed as a normal part of life, and people accepted the fact that death happened; it was much a part of life as birth. Not so long ago, a dying person was always cared for by his family. People tended to die from different types of problems than they do today. For example, so many older people died of pneumonia; it was called the old people's friend. Death from pneumonia was often quick and relatively painless. It might have been a complication of some other disease, which could have taken a longer and a more difficult route. Modern medicine often cures illness and disease, which would have ended in death only a decade or two ago. Today, doctors automatically cure pneumonia with antibiotics, allowing the person to live longer, eventually dying of something else. Death in childbirth used to be common and is now quite rare. Many children died before they reached adulthood: this, too, is rare, and a source of great distress when it does happen, because it seems against all the odds.

The expected life span of men and women has increased dramatically over time, most notably over this last century. Just fifty years ago, organ transplants were unheard of, as was open-heart surgery. We have so many more options today for curing infections, medicines that treat the formally un-treatable, that people's attitude toward health and sickness has dramatically changed. We came to expect cures, and deaths were often viewed as an error, caused by lack of the right treatment. Now death so often happens in hospitals that many people are shielded from it altogether.

Nowadays, we expect doctors can, and will, cure almost anything. So if we are sick, we assume we will be treated and cured. Doctors also expect to be able to cure the patient and many of them view the death of their patient as a personal failure. Most of us grew up in this culture, where we expected the sick to go to hospitals to be returned to health, and we expect treatment to be continued until all possible hope of recovery dies. When death occurs in hospital in this way, both doctor and family may feel that they have failed in some way.

The medical advances and the money available in this country, especially over the last thirty years, has generated a high expectation of being cured, which has contributed to the norm of continuing treatment of the dying man in a hospital environment. The medical approach to end of life care varies a lot with the culture: some cultures retain the attitude that death is but one facet of life.

Now we are so far removed from death, it is much easier to pretend it won't happen, than to face the inevitability of death. When this struggle for survival does go on to the very end, patients die in hospital still attached to machines, and many times alone. Their families bear the hard memories of watching their loved one struggle, and no one has the opportunity to make the most of that critical time to be at peace with loved ones.

Revival of hospice

The concept of hospice is not new, but it had to be revived in a way that this modern culture could accept and see to be a preferable way of dying. Dame Cicely Saunders was the leader in this endeavor in the United Kingdom. As a nurse she had worked with the dying and wanted to make a supported caring approach to death widely available to dying people. She was advised to go to medical school because as a doctor she would have credibility with other doctors, and be more able to influence the medical community. This she did, and she had an enormous impact in England, and through her interactions with medical schools and with doctors, had a large impact in this country, too. She is often described as the founder of modern hospice.

Elisabeth Kubler-Ross was also a prominent direction setter in this country. As a doctor and psychiatrist, teaching in a medical school, she took the unusual tack of interviewing a willing dying patient behind a one-way mirror, in full view and hearing of her medical students. She asked the patient questions about their feelings toward what was happening to them. This was quite revolutionary, as patients had previously been viewed as only the vehicle of interesting problems and diseases.

Dr Ross also gave us a model for understanding the emotional stages a patient typically goes through when they are given a terminal prognosis. The first stage she described as denial and isolation. When patients were first told of their prognosis they were likely to experience shock and disbelief, unable to believe that this was really happening to them. The second stage is anger. The initial phase of disbelief is replaced by feelings of anger, rage, envy, and resentment. That anger may be turned on anyone or anything that irritates or frustrates them. The third stage is bargaining, where the patients may try to negotiate with God, "If I do this or that, please let me recover." When attempts to bargain fail, they typically enter the fourth stage, that of depression. Eventually they come to the fifth stage of acceptance of the prognosis, and begin to do whatever feels right, in the time they have left. Of course the dying person doesn't always move linearly through these steps, and often after accepting the outcome, he relives hope of recovery and returns to denial. We now use this model in many other aspects of life when facing shock or sudden change.

Shifting attitudes of doctors

Dame Saunders and Dr Ross led the way to this new approach in helping the dying, in that they viewed the patient as a whole person, with thoughts, feelings, and emotional needs, and they viewed him as the person best suited to make decisions about his own treatment.

Jerome Groopman, of Beth Israel Deaconess Medical Center and Harvard Medical School, described his experience when he was in medical school on teaching rounds of ward; a patient would be described as a certain disease in bed 10, and another patient would be described as another disease in bed 8, etc.[5] This distancing of a patient, by treating him as a disease rather than as whole person with feelings and emotions, may have helped students avoid dealing with their own feelings. This was typical of medical training at that time. Times are changing, but not as fast as we might hope. Even today, most medical schools programs treat end of life care as a study option and not as a requirement for medical students. In his book, Dr Groopman describes his caring relationships with dying patients, and his teaching from the same perspective.

Today we have so many specialists. It undoubtedly optimizes the depth of understanding and care of specific diseases, but it does have the drawback that patients often talk about feeling abandoned, once the concerned specialist no longer focuses on them, as he recognizes there can be no cure. Patients need to feel loved and supported through all their stages of their illness.

Many doctors are now operating from this primary focus on the dying patient's needs and desires, but many others are still reluctant to accept this focus of caring rather than curing. Lachlan Farrow, the Director of the Palliative Care Program at Beth Israel Deaconess Medical Center, talks to doctors about the kinds of questions doctors need to ask their patients to understand how best to provide support. If a doctor knows how important every last minute is to one patient, when another patient may prefer to focus on quality of life versus heroic measures, then he can make appropriate suggestions about their care. Though he points out once people are enjoying good quality of life, they want more of it. Dr Farrow suggests we call the, Intensive Care Unit in hospitals, the "Intensive Cure Unit," and then when the prognosis is terminal, the patient should be referred to the "Intensive Care Unit." [6]

Fortunately many doctors do practice end of life care in a way that supports the patient and their family. Every hospice has a medical director who takes this approach and acts as an advocate of hospice in his local medical community. In his book *Dying Well*, Ira Byock, M.D., Director of Palliative Care,

Dartmouth-Hitchcock Medical Center, gives tender descriptions of people dying under his hospice care.

Shifting attitudes of patients

An overwhelming proportion of people will say they would choose to die at home, but only about a quarter of that number do, in fact, die at home. In a more recent survey, the percentage dying at home increased slightly. The numbers will never match as people die from accidents or from sudden health crises, but this topic of dying is getting more attention these days.

When a patient and his family are well informed about their options, and well informed about the progression of the disease, the patient can make the best decision about his own treatment. There is no optimal plan that suits everyone, but if the patient, the family, and the doctor are open to discussion, more people will be able to choose how they will spend their last phase of their life for themselves,

Once a person does accept the fact that he is dying, he can begin to put his affairs in order, and choose how he spends the rest of his time and energy. It doesn't mean he is happy to do so; it is usually the most difficult thing he has ever done in his life, but the people who do this can come finally to a peaceful death. This whole process takes time and can't happen if the patient is living in hope of cure until the very last moment.

This is definitely the time people need to take ownership and responsibility for demanding the kind of care they want. That is hard to do unless you have already thought through what you truly want.

Hospice-Like Care

You matter because you are. You matter to the last moment of your life, and we will do all we can, not only to help you die peacefully, but also to live until you die.
—Dame Cicely Saunders, Founder of Modern Hospice

Accepting life expectancy is limited

Coming to the decision to stop chasing a cure may be the hardest thing you ever have to do. Many people leave the decision so long that they only have couple of days before they die. Some never make any decision at all, but they die anyway. When a bereaved person tells me about the illness of their loved one, he so often says, " I wish we had known about hospice sooner." Some people feel guilty later that they pushed their dying loved one into trying to go on, when helping them die peacefully would have felt better in the long run for both of them.

I know from experience in my own family and in other hospice families that there is an alternative to struggling to cure until the end. Some people have been fortunate enough to stand witness to a peaceful, loving ending where the patient himself seems to be a source of love. This experience is still a painful loss of a loved one; however, there is a sense of fulfillment, and the comfort of knowing this was as good as it could have been.

Hospice philosophy

Hospice was based on the premise to help you live until you die, that you live your life to the fullest extent possible for as long as you live. It is really about a way of approaching death that focuses more on the quality of life that you experience toward the end of your life, than chasing the illusive cure. Hospice in the United States provides support for someone dying at home or sometimes in a resident hospice. Sometimes hospice support is provided within a nursing home setting. The philosophy and methodology of hospice, that of comfort care and aggressive pain relief, is becoming a method of care available to everyone no matter where they live. Today, people often come under hospice care only for the last few days of their lives, instead of the months that would have allowed them and their family to come to a more leisurely closure.

Explanation of hospice service

The word "hospice" has become synonymous with "death" and therefore a word and a subject people shy away from. Hospice does nothing to prolong life or to hasten death, but can truly offer patient and families great support over the last few months.

Dame Cicely Saunders founded the first hospice, St Christopher's Inpatient Hospice in London, in 1967. The usual model of hospice in England continues to be special places of residence where dying patients could live and be cared for until they die. In this country today, hospice usually means a team of specialists supporting a patient and his caregiver in their own home. There are some hospice units in hospitals, nursing homes or built for this purpose.

My experience has been with the common form of hospice available across the country, that which supports the dying person in his home. So most of my discussion and my stories relate to this kind of care. The term, hospice, refers to the type of care provided regardless of the location in which it is delivered. Resident hospices are readily available in some parts of the country, most particularly in metropolitan areas.

Hospice care is delivered through a team concept: the patient's regular doctor stays involved, but the hospice team includes a medical director, nurses, home care aides, social workers, spiritual and bereavement coordinators and volunteers. This interdisciplinary team reviews the status of each patient weekly. Different services can be given in the home when needed and desired by the patient and his family. A nurse is assigned to each patient. She will visit or be on call for any questions or problems that come up. Personal care will be provided by the aides in the home each day as needed. A social worker will visit, too, and support the patient and family. If the patient desires, the spiritual coordinator will visit and volunteers can be utilized to give the caregiver a chance for a break. These volunteers are carefully selected and trained by the hospice organization.

In the weekly team meeting, the nurse will talk about the progression of the disease, the symptoms, and the comfort of the patient. The social worker will talk about the family situation and what other help might be needed. The medical director will suggest medication and care changes if needed. The medications are likely to include liquid morphine. Keeping the patient pain free and comfortable is an important goal.

Hospice care also includes bereavement support to the family for twelve months after the death has occurred. This will include calls, mailings, visits and support groups.

Under today's Medicare and insurance company rules, a patient can be under hospice, only if his doctor can declare he is unlikely to live more than six months, and the patient may be asked to sign a "Do Not Resuscitate" form. That can be a hard decision. When are the patient and family ready to accept so clear a definition of the outcome? Palliative care is an intermediate step, under which the patient can receive treatment for symptom control to make them more comfortable, although they are not expected to effect a cure, as well as hospice home care and pain management. Hospices are now also offering palliative care. The patient may be classified as palliative if there is no hope of a cure, although the life expectancy may be longer than six months. Palliative care is more likely to suit people in earlier stages of the dying process. There would be a smooth transition to hospice care when the patient decides to stop pursuing treatments.

Costs

In this country reimbursement for hospice services comes from Medicare, Medicaid, health maintenance organizations and other private insurance plans. If the patient is at home, and requires hospice, any of these plans covers the cost, although some insurance companies' coverage is limited in duration. If the patient needs to be in a nursing facility, Medicare will cover the cost in approved facilities after a qualifying hospital stay. If there is no hospital stay, then Medicare covers the cost after assets have been depleted. In some states, Medicare pays for care in a hospice facility without the qualifying hospital stay. Many hospice agencies offer care on a private-pay, sliding fee scale or charitable basis for those who have insufficient insurance. Speak to your local hospice if you want to pursue one of these options.

Funding for hospice home care covers the cost of the full hospice team: medical director, nurse, home care aides, social worker, spiritual coordinator, volunteers, and bereavement coordinator. The funding also covers costs of medications and needed equipment for the home such as a hospital bed, commode, lift etc. Medicare and insurance companies' funding of palliative care includes the treatments, and services of a doctor, a nurse and home care aides, a social worker and a spiritual coordinator but exclude drugs, and bereavement support.

Ironically this kind of care is not an expensive solution either, compared to the massive amounts of money spent on aggressive care in the last six weeks of life, which account for eighty percent of medical costs. Maybe the health care establishment wants to continue the status quo, because the way of a peaceful death may significantly reduce health care expenditures!

Aggressive pain relief

Hospices have developed excellent models of managing pain. Most of the time they can control the patient's pain. They do leave the patient to make the decision on tradeoffs when being totally free of pain means they would be sleeping more than normal. Some patients choose to keep doing all they can and are willing to accept some pain in order to do that. Hospice nurses very carefully adjust the amount of medication upward so that the patient receives just the right amount to control the pain but not an excess to make them feel "out of it." The timing of pain medication is to suit the patient, not a hospital routine. Addiction may be a concern, but when pain medication is carefully increased to match the demand of the pain, then addiction does not occur. Though it is strange that addiction is an issue when the person is dying.

Benefits

Hospice workers tell many stories of people who were able to come to a resolution of their lives while on hospice care, and die a truly peaceful death. Ninety percent of people say they want to die at home, and hospice care in their own home may be all that's needed. We all deserve to get the supportive loving care at the end of our lives that hospice can provide.

Summary

There are nearly forty million seniors in the US. In the next thirty years that number is expected to double as baby boomers reach age sixty-five. These people are likely to place high importance on dying well just as they have emphasized living well. As more and more discussions are taking place in the media. The topic of death and dying is coming out of the closet.

We should all be entitled to good end of life care, whether we are at home, in a nursing home or in a hospital. It should be hospice-like care, staged to provide palliative treatments, expert pain management, and aggressive comfort care, staffed with doctors, nurses, aides, social workers, volunteers, spiritual and bereavement coordinators and counselors who have chosen to do this work. It has become part of the right to the pursuit of happiness.

Choices

When to choose hospice

A simple answer would be, you choose hospice, because you accept you are dying, and prefer to make the most of the time you have left, rather than to keep trying treatments that no longer provide any benefit. But nothing is simple in this situation.

Daniel Tobin, in his book, Peaceful Dying, gives a detail set of steps for people to follow. He describes this as a step-by-step guide to preserving your dignity, your choice, and your inner peace at the end of life.

Everyone is different, and each of us is likely to have a different outlook at different phases of our lives. Someone in her early thirties, with young children, is in a very different situation than a much older woman, who may feel she has fulfilled all she needed to do in life, and naturally her choice of treatment is likely to be different. Most people choose treatment until their doctor says there is nothing more to be done, except to make sure you are as comfortable as possible. Some doctors acknowledge this far sooner than others. Some prefer to keep the hope of recovery open until the last moment.

As a patient's illness progress and curative treatments do

less and less good, he may choose to focus on the quality of life and controlling symptoms, rather than going through possibly futile curative procedures. Doctors often assume that their patient will want more and more aggressive curative treatments, and may not immediately think of the palliative or hospice care option. Some people with advanced heart disease, lung disease, cancer or other serious illness, chose to stay home with the support of a palliative or hospice care team as opposed to returning to the hospital during flare-ups. Even that picture is less simple today, as some medications make keep hope of recovery alive until quite close to the end.

Palliative and hospice care focus on supporting and maximizing your quality of life for as long as you are living. The focus shifts from curing to caring, treating a person to keep them comfortable in the setting of their choice. It gives the patient and his family time to deal with psychological and spiritual pain, at the same time as their physical symptoms are monitored and relieved.

Planning ahead

If people think ahead about how they will want to be treated and talk to their loved ones about their wishes, the whole process will be much easier when such decisions are needed. Older people may be very clear that they want to maintain a good quality of life, and heroic treatments at the end of a long and fruitful life are the last thing they want. Some people say they want to die suddenly, so they don't have to think about it, or to suffer treatment or pain. An emergency room nurse said a three day warning is about right—giving people time to say goodbye to their loved ones, which lessens the burden of grief on the remaining family and friends. In hospice, we often see a dying person and his family for much longer than that before he dies, and we see that the extra time allows both the patient and his loved ones to say all they have to say to each other.

Some people are very reluctant to talk about death. This is usually because people can't bear to think of leaving or losing loved ones. Still, it is much easier to talk about a potential death when you are talking about something that may be way into the future. The "Five Wishes Document"[4] is a useful vehicle for raising the questions that need answers. It asks questions about how you would like to be treated in different situations. How we answer these questions may change over time, as we age, and as we get sicker.

Identifying a health care proxy is also important. Your designated health care proxy is the person who will speak on your behalf should you be unable to do so. More hospitals are requiring a designated health care proxy for the duration of a patients stay in hospital.

I know I was so glad that I had talked with my mother ahead of her final illness. I could talk quite clearly with the doctor when he needed to discuss options for her treatment. I knew the answers she would have given had she been able to respond. So she was treated how she preferred, and I suffered no guilt by guessing what she would have said. I knew.

Choosing hope

When a person is dying, there is often a conspiracy around her. The doctor may feel he wants to leave her with the hope that she will recover. Her family may also join the conspiracy because they want to believe she will recover. It is also magical thinking: if we believe hard enough, it will make it so. So people hold onto the concept that if they keep hope for a cure, there is still a chance it will happen. Yes, miracles do occur. But usually the outcome of this sort of thinking is that the dying person struggles with more and more treatments, doesn't have the opportunity to be with loved ones in her own home and finally dies in hospital, maybe alone and still hooked up to machines.

If we accept death is coming, all hope is not lost. We just have to adjust our hopes. We cannot hope to live forever, because it's obviously impossible. The hopes of the dying person need to be tailored to his immediate situation. If he is still mobile, he may hope to spend time visiting his favorite places and his favorite people. He may hope to make the very most of his time with his loved ones. He may hope to close old wounds, he may hope for reconciliation, and he may hope for visits from many old friends.

When the focus is on health, his hope will be to be kept comfortable, to be free of pain. He may hope to be surrounded by caring, loving people, in a well-loved environment. He may hope of being at peace, of passing from this world serenely, to the divine place of his personal vision.

Choosing a hospice

There is a Federation of Hospice and Palliative Care in most states, and they will share a complete listing of hospices. The majority of hospices nationwide is certified by Medicare, and must be licensed by the state. Most hospices also maintain membership in the National Hospice and Palliative Care Organization, which encourages a sharing of ideas and solutions at the national level. Recently, many hospices seek accreditation from the Joint Commission on the Accreditation of Healthcare Organizations, which operates to further ensure quality care,

The dying person can receive hospice or palliative care whether they are at home, in a nursing home, or in a hospice facility. If you choose to have hospice care in your home, you will have to choose a hospice willing to visit homes in your area. You still may have two or three choices.

Patient choice

I am well aware that I haven't answered my own question, which was when to choose hospice. It is still the patient's choice, and that's how it should be. If each of us has thought about these issues ahead of time, and acknowledges death as a part of life, we are more likely to be able to make a choice of hospice in good time, so that we can spend our final days in the setting of our choice, surrounded by people we love.

Coming to Closure on a Lifetime

How can I learn to dance with a terminal illness? The moment that you ask that question the orchestra is already tuning up. Your willingness to explore is the dance. Your willingness to seek is the finding. The minute you say, "There is another way to do this," you have found the other way. Trust the portion of you from where the question came. Honor it above all illusion of living and dying in illness—and your dance has begun.

—*From Emmanuel's Book II,* by Pat Rodegast and Judith Stanton. [7]

Moving
to Acceptance

Coming to accept death is the first stage in the business of dying. The doctor may have been very clear that there is no hope of a cure, but one day the patient feels he can become resigned to this fact and the next day he hears of some new, potential cure and starts hoping all over again. Occasionally some people do pull through and recover from an ominous diagnosis. Some never do come to accept that they will die shortly and they die anyway. Usually when the patient and family have accepted the fact death is imminent and prepare as best they can, the death itself tends to be more peaceful. So how does anybody come to accept the fact that they will die sooner rather than later? At what point in an illness does someone decide the effort to continue treatment is futile and may even be worse than the disease? What are our fears? What is our belief system? Again, the answer, as well as the experience, is going to be unique for each individual.

If we believe in a life after death that will be beautiful perhaps it's a little easier to accept the end of this life, but our ties to people here becomes a huge impediment in this process. The patient loves them and doesn't want to leave them. They are concerned about how well their loved ones will be able to cope without them. There is the pull of the future they had planned.

Some people get a clear message from their doctor and come to an acceptance of the fact of their imminent death, quickly. Others continue their fight for life right on to their deathbed.

Barbara

One day at work I met Barbara, a woman I had not seen for a couple of years, although we had worked together closely in the past, then we had shared a strong mutual respect and similar values. I had heard from someone that she had been quite ill. She looked terrible. She had lost weight, her skin was drawn tightly across her skull and her skin was white.

When she saw me Barbara called my name and rushed to me. I opened my arms and hugged her for the first time. I felt a surge of energy go through me to her, though I still didn't know what was wrong. She sat down and told me of her battle with cancer, her hopes and her fears. I just listened, and that was all she needed. She recounted all the steps she had already been through, the different stages of her illness and the various treatments she had been given. Then she talked about her fears for the future, saying " I don't know if I'm going to make it," and moved on to describe her family and how well they would or would not cope without her. Her main concern was how her daughter would manage without her. Furthermore, she was grieving for the future events in her daughter's life that she would never share.

Barbara died a couple of months after our meeting. I reviewed our conversation and realized I had been hearing her process of coming to acceptance of her own impending death. As Barbara talked, laying it all out for me and explaining the details, she was beginning to recognize and accept what was happening to her. Before she died, she had been able to put her affairs in order, she made provision for her family and completed whatever she felt she needed to do

This latter phase is so incredibly difficult for everyone. We can't tell how we will cope until we are faced with an identical situation. People who do get a clear message from their doctors are the ones who are more likely to be able to come to terms with death sooner and choose to use their remaining time with whomsoever is most important to them.

Martha

A hospice nurse told me the following story: it is about the experience she had when she went to visit an elderly woman, Martha, to explain to her and her family just what hospice would and wouldn't be able to do to help make her last months comfortable. The patient and family agreed to accept hospice support and signed on. The two daughters left the room so that Martha could talk privately with the nurse in case she had any more questions.

Martha said to the nurse, "Now you're the Kevorkian people aren't you? I want out quickly." The nurse responded by explaining that hospice was about helping people be as comfortable as possible and would not do anything to speed up the time of death.

This was not what Martha wanted to hear. She was angry about being in her situation, previously she had been quite a dominating force in her family. Her husband had died years earlier and her daughters were tired of trying to keep her happy when nothing was good enough for her. One daughter continued to be thoughtful and caring even though she was subjected to verbal abuse. Martha had a difficult disease that caused pain which couldn't be fully relieved during its progression over the course of three or four months.

The nurse continued her daily visits and one day Martha said to her, "I know what this dying is about. The point of my being ill for this time is so that I can learn not to be nasty and to be grateful to my family for their support and love."

Martha truly changed during this time and managed to establish more loving relationships with her family. In the end, her last days were quite peaceful and she died with her family around her. Even after she had gone, there was a difference in the relationships between and amongst all the family members: they had become closer and more intimate then they had ever been before. Possibly Martha had articulated the purpose of the dying process, which was so that she could learn to be a pleasant person.

Summary

Coming to acceptance may be the hardest part of all in the process of dying. How do we decide how long we should pursue treatment? When the loved ones see the patient clinging to every hope of a cure it is very hard to disillusion them.

Simultaneously, family and friends struggle themselves. They may believe that holding on to hope is the right thing to do. Coming to acceptance may be a quick or a very lengthy process, or it may not happen at all. In either case it does seem to need to happen if the patient is going to go through the steps of dying, move through this final stage of growth in order to finalize their life, and die a peaceful death.

The Business of Dying

Once the patients and the key people in their lives can acknowledge to themselves and to each other the certainty that this life is really coming to an end, they can face what is needed to prepare for the work of dying. Dr Byock expressed this business of dying as a series of steps. The business of dying is to finalize an individual's lifetime: it is to say I'm sorry, forgive me, I've forgiven you, thank you, I love you, and goodbye. In essence:

Acknowledge the wrongs done to you and forgive those who perpetuated the wrongdoing.
Acknowledge the wrongs you have done to others, say sorry, and ask for forgiveness.
Say thank you to others who have helped you in life,
Say I love you.

Witnessing the process
When I sat with a patient as a volunteer, I would ask

questions about his life. Often he would enjoy telling me about good memories and different events in his life. Talking about these memories seemed to help him bring events in his life together, he was able to see how the pieces of his life fitted together: they were no longer incomprehensible, random hotchpotch events. Sometimes those memories were not too pleasant, and a patient might be relieved to talk about them. Another patient clearly held some memories secret. Those unshared secrets, or even family-held secrets, often seemed to be a source of suffering for him as for example, were the following patients.

Joseph

Joseph had had a difficult life and responded to his pain by abusing alcohol. His relationship with his son had never evolved from much shared unhappiness in their past. As Joseph was dying, his son filled all the basic requirements of a hospice caretaker, taking care of all Joseph's physical needs, but much of the time the dying patient was alone and struggling with physical and emotional pain.

Grace

Grace had never been expressive about love and caring. Her husband was in such emotional pain that they could not even make a connection on her deathbed. She was very pleasant with me and appreciative of my help, but would turn her head away from her husband. I didn't know their history, but I do know she was in pain for days as she fought to hold onto this world.

Now I've seen sufficient situations to find a clear difference between the patients moving through whatever emotional growth was needed and bridging the gaps with loved ones, and the patients with unfinished emotional business who, as a result, were more likely to suffer and struggle at the end of their life. When the emotional past has been put to rest a startling intimacy between the family members can develop and their love for each other is palpable.

Forgive and ask forgiveness

Sometimes the conversations I had with patients would lead us to topics of forgiveness: we were able to identify business to which the patient needed to attend. Some of the first steps seem to be righting the perceived wrongs of a lifetime, of being able to say sorry and ask forgiveness, of being able to forgive and let go of grievances.

Many hospice patients show signs of anxiety that appears to be connected to an event they regret or can't resolve. Further examples, which convince me of this need for forgiveness, include the following. A hospice nurse told me of a patient who was muttering on her deathbed. Her impression was that there were, within the context of these mumblings, memories of child abuse. Plainly the patient was haunted by the fact that she could not, did not, or was not able to prevent abuse. A divorced man was estranged from his children of his first marriage and cried and cried over their loss, although his disease prevented him from articulating or resolving the conflict. Another woman tried hard to find "the baby." It transpired that she had had her baby die at birth. That death had been a secret from the rest of her children, something that she had not been able to talk about for years. Such unresolved and secret issues as these might sit heavily on our conscience. Often it is just ourselves we have to forgive, we need to acknowledge and accept that we did the best we could at the time. However, it seems to be harder for people who cannot share their feelings with others and try to carry their secret burdens to the grave. Frequently people do tell a story to someone, then feel free of it and are able to let it go.

The majority of people, who work around the dying, believe in an afterlife. All the hospice workers I've talked to certainly do and the families who stayed close to their dying loved ones usually do so, too. Most see the end as something special, light, and loving. Only once did I hear of a dying man who looked terrified as if he had found hell as he died. That was a man who had many things to feel guilty about in his life. He had grown up with a belief in heaven and hell, and he must have expected to find hell. Maybe we find just what we expect to find. If he had forgiven himself, he would have been at peace with himself, and accepted that he gave of his best in his lifetime. I am convinced that is enough. None of us has been perfect! The only thing I can believe in is love.

Those amongst us who have performed horrendous acts of violence in adulthood usually learned such behavior when very small children, we did what we needed to do to protect the child within. Everyone can turn their lives around, by feeling deeply sorry for the act, the ill brought to others, and by forgiving themselves.

Rifts occur in all kinds of families. A dying parent may regret the fact that he hasn't seen a son in thirty years. He might be able to bring himself to write a letter to beg forgiveness, and offer his own forgiveness. We in hospice have seen many reunions of estranged family members as someone is dying. In many cases the hospice nurse and social worker have been able to assist by facilitating a family meeting where some issues get resolved. In addition, nurses and social workers will also encourage people to write letters to express their feelings, if desirable they will even write a letter dictated by a patient. Frequently we have seen the adult children lay aside old wounds and come together at the dying parent's bedside. Sometimes these reunions are both joyous and tearful; occasionally they are constrained by old resentments or resurfacing ones—the very issues that drove them apart in the first place.

Sometimes one person tries to make amends but the other refuses to let go of the old hurts. It has been known for the second party to have died, or have no known address or other circumstances have prevented resolution. There is no magic remedy here. If the patient can fully acknowledge and understand the impact of his action and be truly sorry, he can forgive himself. The act of forgiveness makes an internal shift in the person doing the forgiving, this helps the patient let go, even if the forgiveness is not reciprocated in a way he wants to see.

Another example of a family coming together and forgetting old antagonisms made an unforgettable impression on me. I cannot even tell you what happened in the room, but something within the family changed and the father died peacefully quite shortly afterward.

Paul

As a volunteer, I was sent to a hospice patient in a nursing home. It was clear that I had been sent to aid the family as the patient, Paul, had end stage Alzheimer's and was not consciously aware of my presence. At the doctor's suggestion, the strong-minded son had made the decision to withhold some medication, which would mean his father's death would occur within days. The old man was agitated and tried fruitlessly to communicate. Paul's son and his wife had been at the bedside all day not wanting to even leave for one moment even to get a meal, they were determined to ensure that there was no risk of Paul dying alone.

I introduced myself to the son and his wife and asked a few questions about their father's life. They were so happy to share their memories and pulled out a photograph album to show me some of their history. Once they were comfortable with me, they decided to go get a meal and leave me with Paul.

After they left, I asked quietly for help for this patient. I don't call it prayer, though some might. I told his higher self to pay attention because this human being was getting ready to come over and needed some help. I sat quietly and basked in the light and love that poured into his room. The old man became calm and slept peacefully.

The son and his wife returned, and shortly afterward Paul's two daughters arrived. The son explained his decision to withhold medication. One of his sisters was clearly furious and you could see the long pattern of their strained interaction. I can't remember what I said, and the words I used do not really matter. I think it was just the energy in the room transformed the situation and very shortly the siblings were able to accept that the end for Paul was close. They were able to hug one another and cry together.

I took my leave of them, and each of those four adults stood up and hugged me and thanked me profusely for "caring about their father."

In some way, this family was able to set aside its own battles together as their father left this life. Perhaps he was leaving them with his final gift, which was to reunite the family in peace. I personally felt I couldn't have spent two hours in any more profitable way, even though I didn't understand what I had done.

Conversely I have known a patient hold on to life by a thread in the hope of reconciliation, and his dream does not come to fruition. Some hold onto their grievances to the very end. Hospice workers can explain what is happening to family members and encourage them to help the patient write a letter. Thus the patient is able to dictate his offerings of love, forgiveness and in return request forgiveness. Even if those letters are never answered, the act of being clear and articulating his feelings, enables the patient to free himself of his emotional burden.

Practical affairs

Preparing for the end involves practical matters. Important steps include getting the finances in order: making sure the will is current and paperwork prepared, perhaps teaching his spouse the skills she will need to manage on her own. Leaving the practical things in good order allows people to rest and is a real gift to those who will be left with the burden of coping when they are least able to do so. Most people who are dying are very concerned about their loved ones' ability to cope without them. If they can talk through issues and put their own affairs in good order it makes it easier for the patient to let go. Basic things such as finishing a project, tidying personal affairs, and giving away items like jewelry to a favorite grandchild may be very important to the dying patient.

Often the patient helps plan his own funeral and lets people know his wishes about whether to be buried or cremated, and where, and which funeral director to use. When such arrangements are made it does relieve the burden on his loved ones who would otherwise be faced with these decisions at a vulnerable time when they would be least able to cope with them. At best they might feel unsure of what the patient would have wanted. In each case it is better to discuss the patient's wishes and the manner of his departure when he is well, then details can be discussed rationally and made clear to the family, but that is not always what has been done.

Living life to the fullest

There is a lot of living to be crammed into those final weeks and months before death occurs. If possible, do the things one loves one more time: the travel you perhaps never had time for, or the visits that can't be delayed any longer. We hear news items about organizations granting wishes for dying children, but many family and friends rally around to do the same for those they care about.

So there may be places to visit for one last time, things to do for a last time, people to see. Incredibly knowing time may be so limited focuses the mind on what is truly important. This is what maximizing quality of life is all about. This is how we should live all the time. We should focus on that which is truly important.

Roger

Despite taking some prescribed experimental chemotherapy in the hope that he would give himself a little longer to live, Roger knew he was dying because his doctors had been very clear about his having less than a year to live. He accepted this reality but still he wanted to fill the time he had left with the people and activities he had loved all his life. He had fulfilled his national service as a pilot and had always wanted to fly in a small plane again. Two of his good friends arranged to take him up in a small plane so he could relive that experience one last time. In addition he had also loved to sail his own boat from port to port for three weeks each summer. He wanted to do it again, though he was too weak to tackle it alone. Five other people rallied around: some sailing the boat over the long passages, some just aiding and standing by, another driving to collect more chemo at the right time. Less than a week from his death his son took him shopping in a wheelchair, so he could buy jewelry for his daughters-in-law to remember him by. He was only bed ridden for 3 or 4 days before he died. He truly had made the most of his last 10 months.

This man had come to accept the inevitability of his death quite soon after the diagnosis was given. The doctors had helped by being very clear he had only months to live. He made the very most of the time he had left to live. He took care of business and finances. He took care of his family. He left with no issues of forgiving undone. He had said I love you, and goodbye.

Waiting for a special event

Many people who are dying can hold onto life until something special happens. Clara looked forward to the birth of her great granddaughter and once she had seen her, died peacefully a few days later. Bill, wanted to be able to celebrate his 50th wedding anniversary with his wife, he died a couple of weeks afterward. Someone in my own family waited until her granddaughter returned from a long trip so that she could see her well and happy before she died. Key element of their lives came to completion for these patients, and then it was appropriate for them to die.

Leaving children

It must be incredibly difficult to go through the process of letting go of your attachment to life, but even worse must be to die knowing you are leaving a family of young children. You would be worried both about their being loved and cared for adequately, and about them remembering you. Some people have made special things themselves for each child as a keepsake and memory holder. One young woman made a special photo album for each child with photos of herself with the child at each stage of their lives. Others have written a journal, to be given to the child later, or made a video for their child in which they have recorded themselves speaking to the child of their love, and giving them advice for life.

Priscilla

I loved to visit Priscilla who was dying at home: she was being cared for by her son. The son had had a struggle in some phases of his life, but was now an adult, living with his mother.

The dying mother cried one day and shared with me how concerned she was for her son and wondered how well he would cope once she was dead. We talked about it and I asked about the extended family and other support. Priscilla could see that there really was a lot of family support and people who would rally around to help her son. The son, too, really grew emotionally during the whole process and was a great support to his mother, even though others in the family hadn't thought he would be able to sustain her in her illness. Moreover, Priscilla also shared her fears about her son with the rest of the family and a sister was able to reassure her that they would be there to support him.

Gradually Priscilla came to see that her son would be able to cope without her and that he would have some good support from others in the family. That was part of her being ready to let go.

Lucy and Bette

I visited Lucy a week after her mother died. She had been very close to her mother and right up until the last few days before her death she hadn't been able to accept that her mother was going to die. Two months earlier the hospice nurse had suggested that Lucy tell Bette that it was okay to die. Even though Lucy said the words to her mother, in her heart she wasn't to say them sincerely ready to let her mother go. She became her caretaker and spent nearly all her time looking after her mother and talking to her. Many times Bette described events and experiences to Lucy in her process of dying. Lucy said some people thought Bette was rambling in her comments, but Lucy said she could understand most of them. Here are some of the things Lucy described.

One day Bette talked about seeing the connectedness of everything. She would point out things in her room, such as a chair, a picture, a wall and say they were all connected, part of each other, part of the same energy.

She began to see people that no one else could see. In the past she had called herself such a good Catholic that she didn't have to go to church. She saw priests around her and could clearly describe their colorful robes. Lucy wondered whether she was seeing her own funeral or the reception committee waiting in the next world. Another time Bette saw relatives who had died: she knew they were waiting for her and that they would be greeting her when she left this life.

Bette had become curled to one side after surgery and could not sit up by herself. She was sleeping one day, in this position, when suddenly she sat up and started talking about what she had just seen.

Several times Bette seemed comatose for a day or two. Once Lucy felt she was really leaving and she grabbed her and called out, "Mommy, don't leave me!" That time Bette opened her eyes and looked at Lucy. Later she was able to talk about what she had experienced. Bette said she had moved into a peaceful place that was filled with a wondrous light and she knew she was dying. She heard herself called back and said she was glad that she had a little longer with her family.

The family felt that they had been on a deathwatch for two months as they watched Bette fade and return repeatedly. The hospice nurse and aides also thought she was about to die several times. At times Lucy felt this was not her mother as she saw as the renewed strength returned. This woman had managed to tap into some incredible strength to hang on until she felt her daughter and other family members were going to be strong enough to cope with her death and their new life alone.

Lucy's father had come to accept the fact his wife was dying several months before Lucy. It was Lucy who couldn't come to terms with it. The mother was sharing her approach to death and was able to help Lucy see and understand what was happening. Her mother was at peace with her religious beliefs, and gave Lucy a sense of there being something more than this life's experiences, this helped Lucy to come to accept her mother's need to let go.

Evelyn

Another hospice patient had been less than an ideal spouse. She and her husband had been divorced twenty years earlier after some altercations. Toward the end of her life Evelyn's ex-husband had taken her back to his home to care for her. Initially the relationship was very difficult and fraught with past anger. The hospice nurse had joked that she often wondered what she would find each time she went into the home. Eventually those two individuals made peace with their past and with each other. Even after she died, the husband grieved for not only his ex-wife's death, but also the previous twenty years when they had not been together and at peace.

Getting permission to leave

Even when the dying person has accepted the reality of his

dying, family and friends may not be able to do so. One woman in one of my bereavement groups told me of her own guilt at pushing her dying husband into trying yet one more treatment because she wasn't ready to accept the fact that he was dying. Talking openly with one another can alleviate this situation because pain and tears are shared.

There are some wonderful stories of a dying child expressing their concern that his parents will not be able to cope with the grief when he goes. When the parent comes to peace the child dies quite quickly.

So this is another major reason why a person holds onto life as long as possible, even though he may be suffering. That patient may die very shortly, even minutes, after their loved one says, "I will be OK, you can go now."

When my own mother was in hospital, I knew she didn't have long to live, although the doctors hadn't yet diagnosed what was wrong with her. At one point she said to me, "Life is too much trouble." I was able to reply, "Yes, it's too much trouble and you can give up the struggle now, and leave."

I was making my regular first phone call to a surviving son of a hospice patient, and he told me of an experience he had had the night before his mother's death. Up to that point he had been very reluctant to accept the fact that his mother was dying and kept hoping for a miraculous cure for her. He told me, "I was lying awake, thinking about her and the way she was suffering, and I just knew in my heart it was OK for her to leave now. She needed to die and I didn't want to hold onto her seeing her suffer like this. As soon as I felt that in my heart I saw her clearly in front of me with a golden halo, then I knew she would be all right."

His mother died early the next morning. He felt at peace and very comforted by the fact that he had been able to come to understand his dilemmas so let her go peacefully.

Dementia patients

Preparing for death for patients with Alzheimer's or dementia is devoid of understanding of these above steps. I have seen such patients struggle to grasp and understand what is happening to them for so long, then they come to peace only in the last few days or weeks of their illness. Some of them seem to understand things we don't see, and even express a perspective that's intriguing. I have wondered whether they are performing a service on an astral level, then they get stuck there and cannot get out it—that is, either back into "normal" reality or released into death. We do seem to have to be in our body before we can leave it.

Emily

When first I went to visit Emily, an Alzheimer's patient in her 90s, she took my hands and said, "Ah, maybe it's you! You are the one who has come to show me the way." Emily's daughter rolled her eyes, but I knew what Emily meant, although I didn't know if I knew how to do what she asked.

When I was with Emily, I found she responded to my unspoken wish. If I wanted her to calm down, I'd be very grounded and calm, and in my mind tell her to sit down now and be calm. Her energy would mirror mine and she'd be calm and sit down. Although Emily would get very upset and panicky as she tried to follow other people's conversations and couldn't, she often talked to me in a reasonably coherent way as long as I let her lead and gave very simple answers to her questions. I didn't try to say anything to her unless she led. She responded positively to tacit attention. If I just sat with her silently and offered her love she would be quite calm. She taught me quite clearly when I missed the point. It was not for me to try to encourage her to do anything as one would a child.

On another occasion Emily took my arm and said, "Maybe it's today that you are going to show me the way." She faded quite slowly up until the last week or two and then seemed to accept that the end was coming and deteriorated quite quickly.

Alice

My aunt Alice was in a nursing home because she was stricken with senile dementia. I hadn't been able to visit her for several years. I managed the 3000 miles to visit my mother annually, but I didn't take the extra two days to visit an aunt who everyone assured me would not recognize me. My mother was listed as next of kin, but she was no longer able to make the journey to visit her sister, both because of the physical stress of the journey and because she had found her last visit emotionally overwhelming.

I kept thinking about that aunt, for no apparent reason for several weeks, so I wrote to the nursing home; eventually a reply came to say that she had become terribly confused and they had had to move her to another facility. The authorities had neglected to inform my mother of my aunt's move, therefore my mother was in ignorance of her beloved sister's whereabouts.

A year or two later I made the trip to visit my aunt in the new nursing home because my mother was no longer able to visit her: in a sense I was going for both of us. I met with the home manager and then a nurse took me into the day room to meet my aunt.

The nurse tried to rouse my aunt saying, "Alice, your niece from America is here." Alice looked straight at me and said, "How's my sister?" It had been 6 or 7 years since she recognized anyone, so the nurse was astounded that she knew me well enough to ask about my mother. As I sat with Alice for a few hours, she lapsed in and out of her own world. As I started to take my leave, she said, "I'm coming with you. I need to be with you because you know." However, I said, "Goodbye," and started my trip back. At the end of the day, one half of my body felt totally exhausted, as if I was 95. Then I realized Alice had come with me energetically. "Alice," I said, " Get out of my body and back into your own." I immediately I felt the fatigue leave me and I was back to my forty-something self.

A couple of years later my mother died. I realized that she would be able show her sister, my aunt "the way." Now she would be able to help her sister over to the other side. I wrote to the nursing home saying my mother had died and I expected something to happen to Alice shortly and asked to be kept informed, as I was next of kin. The return mail disclosed that Alice had died just a few weeks after her sister. The letter concluded that my aunt's last few days had been very peaceful.

Both Aunt Alice and Emily floated in and out of any kind of thought process. They both knew they needed help to figure out how to die. They were lost in their own world and knew it. Their energy seemed out on the astral plane. The connection I was able to form with them, joining them, which was to join them where they were, aided their process of communication with me: it put them at their ease with me and helped bridge a vital gap which created the right conditions for a little, relatively normal, behavior. Emily "gave up" and accepted she was dying about 3 weeks before she died. Alice struggled until the last few days when she came to peace and let go.

Bernard

A friend's husband, Bernard, also took eight years to die of Alzheimer's. I found he was receptive to communication in the same way as Emily and Alice had been. He replied to my simple question on the phone once with a cohesive answer, a good eighteen months after anyone thought he was capable of doing so. My friend tried similar techniques of modeling and giving directions in her mind, to her husband, and found them helpful.

Coming to peace
The process of coming to peace was a much longer one for my mother than for my father. My father died when I was 40. The event triggered my own mid life crisis and growth. It was only after I had come to understand myself a good deal better that I was capable of being anywhere near people who were dying. My mother was 77 at the time of her husband's death and was to die ten years after him. During the last seven years of her life I was able to visit her at least annually, even once a quarter for 2-3 years. We talked frequently on the phone, too. Therefore, during those years we talked about life and death: of our interdependent life histories and her view of how she wanted to die. Always she was a person who enjoyed being with and helping others. At the same time she would complain about the trials of her life, current and past, and worry about the details of living alone.

When we talked about dying my mother was absolute that she did not want to be ill for a long time. She hoped never to go into a nursing home and expressed her desire to be in her own home until she was, "Carried out in a pine box." She had a weak heart from the time she was a teenager and had many minor heart attacks during her lifetime. Latterly her sight worsened until she became legally blind. Still she could cope alone in a warden assisted retirement home.

I talked to her about masters in the far east, the Buddhists monks of whom it was said, could announce they were going to die, then sit and meditate until they did so. I postulated that we have to stay in our bodies until we have learned something we need to learn. So if we have done our work of growth and learning ahead of time while we were still fit, then perhaps we, too, could pass over without needing to be ill for a long time.

We continued to talk about these things over a period of several years. I taught her to meditate, so that she could be less anxious about her problems. Then on another visit, I shared with her my experience with my deceased father's spirit, which I had in a meditation group. It was then that I learned that there had been mediums in the family. Was it possible that I was carrying on a family tradition? I asked myself. One day I led her in meditation and told her to ask her guardian angel to come to her. We both felt a peaceful presence. I suggested she ask for her guardian angel's presence and guidance when she went to bed each night, and ask him, or her, for help in letting go and clearing out anything she needed to. Such learning as was needed, I reasoned, could go on while she was sleeping.

For several nights she woke up crying. When she told me this on the phone, I said, " That's wonderful, you are letting go of sadness." "Oh yes," she said, "I have had a very sad life." This old lady slowly became much happier. I would hear her complain less often. Even photos of her changed dramatically. Always before she had avoided having her photo taken and would frown at the camera. She began looking lighter and lighter, happier and happier. I have a beautiful photo of her, taken with my daughter, just nine months before she died.

Once she said to me, "You think about me a lot, I know." Another time, when I had just returned from a visit and had a restless night still thinking about her, she said, "I got up in the night to make tea, and you were in the living room, I could feel your presence." I was glad she could feel our closeness and support even though I was 3,000 miles away.

All this time she continued to help others. By now she was 86, legally blind, but still very interested in and concerned about other people; she insisted on being driven to church early in order to help the poor old folks. She still visited people in a nursing home and at Christmas gave a vote of thanks to the staff. I had a wonderful visit with her when I visited in the spring before she died.

A few months after my return from England, my mother developed a lung infection. She was treated at home for two weeks, by a visiting nurse. I telephoned each day and talked to both my mother and my brother who lived nearby. My brother telephoned me one Monday morning, saying, "Mother is worse and I'm waiting for the doctor, I think you should come now.

The doctor arrived, diagnosed pneumonia and admitted her to hospital that afternoon. I flew across the Atlantic that night and walked into her hospital room by 8 a.m. the next morning.

I stayed at her side for the next four days. She started having strange turns as her heartbeat was erratic. The doctor pulled me aside and asked whether I would want her resuscitated if her heart stopped. Without hesitation I replied. "No, do not resuscitate. She and I have talked about her death, I know this is what she would want." I stopped the planned X-ray and tests. As she had those odd turns she responded to my voice. By this time the consultant suspected she had a major invasion of cancer.

I sat calmly at her side for four days, holding her hand. She became calm. Her open eyes, took up multiple levels of not seeing. At one point an intense golden light shone out from her pupils and I felt an old recognition of a soul I had known for eons. I was torn between not wanting to tell anyone in case they thought I was crazy, and wanting to ask if anyone else could see it, too. The light only lasted a few seconds, so I had no time to seek confirmation.

I still wonder whether my mother's work on letting go of some of the issues and distractions in her life, helped her die without being ill for too long. I was comforted by the fact that she had died the death she had wanted, and that I had been there and had clearly been of some help to her.

Sudden death

When people die suddenly there is no time to go through the normal processes of coming to the acceptance of imminent death. After the death has occurred some of the survivors can piece together certain, albeit random, events, which seem to indicate that the person was unconsciously getting ready to die.

Kathleen

I had worked closely with Kathleen at work. She was part of a committee that oversaw the work for which I was responsible. We had had a similar outlook on the world and work, and she had been in an ideal position to give me support in the job I was doing. Occasionally I would go to see her to have an hour's discussion about achievements at work and new goals.

Two weeks before Kathleen died, I spent time with her and we had an odd interaction. She said, "We hired you to do x, you did it, thank you. We hired you to do y, you did it, thank you. We hired you to do z, you did it, thank you." It is rare for someone to thank you like that. I thanked her for all her support, and I felt a strange exchange of energy as I said goodbye.

Kathleen died of a heart attack two weeks later. As I relived our earlier meeting and conversation, the mystery began to make sense. I felt we had completed our relationship and were effectively saying goodbye. At some level she knew she was leaving this life and she had completed her business with me. Later I talked to two friends who had had similar connections with her prior to her death. Like me, they had met Kathleen during the last two weeks of her had similar conversations with her.

Kevin

I talked to Amy, whose husband Kevin had died suddenly of a heart attack. While Amy mused over events that occurred just before Kevin died, she could see a pattern emerge.

Amy's husband of twenty years had been struggling with certain aspects of his job. He was tremendously outgoing and caring, but was beginning to live with a great burden. He was open and trusting, however many of the people he had helped had let him down. Meanwhile, Amy was also pregnant and, although Kevin was saying all the right words, he was not wholeheartedly embracing the idea of being a father in his late forties.

Amy pondered over these signs a year later, she surmised that he had really done as much of his work here as he could do and then his purpose in being here was over.

Summary

In the dying process, people do undergo significant changes, the words, the" final stage of growth" seem very apt. People do ask forgiveness, they do accept others in ways they never had before, and they do come to terms with who they are and accept it. When all the baggage of a lifetime is released, they can celebrate life and rejoice in the love that surrounds them and in the love that flows through them.

Such conclusions are profoundly touching, full of love and sorrow, they play again and again in our minds. Sad yes, but beautiful, with a strong sense that this is as good as life gets.

Family Reconciliations and Interactions with the Dying

Each of our lives takes many twists and turns. Usually, each of us experience good times and tough times, joyful times and painful times. It seems to be the nature of living. It is also so easy to be so busy, especially in this country, and in this time, that we are barely conscious of what is happening around us. We miss so many opportunities to be truly present for someone who wanted our attention.

Sometimes forgiveness needs to be addressed, although in many cases such issues were resolved long ago.

Forgiving others
Often we manage to be terribly nice with strangers or co-

workers, and take our fatigue and exasperation home with us. It is so easy for each of us to blame the other people in our lives for things that go wrong. It is true that we all carry some burden and some carry far greater burdens than others. However, we don't change our own lives until we stop the blaming and take responsibilities for our own actions. There may have been events in our lives where people did us great injustice, and the younger we were, when these events occurred, the harder it is to change the behaviors we learned to affect, in order to cope with our situations.

Forgiving is not a big benevolent act. If we think we are being big hearted or magnanimous that we are good enough to forgive, we aren't really forgiving at all. Forgiving is quite a selfish act. You set yourself free. Those resentments and angry memories erode at our own peace and happiness. Then the biggest benefit is that if we truly forgive someone else, it loses its hold on us, and we don't even need a thank you from the other person.

I know I have been slow to forgive. In my head I can say all the right things, but my heart holds onto hurting history. I have let years pass without being aware that I was still holding a grudge against someone. My way of release is to go into the hurt within me and just hold onto it, let it intensify, until suddenly it is gone. Other people will have their own processes.

This kind of unfinished business can be very disturbing to someone who is dying. Dying peacefully requires the dying person to truly be at peace. So if he still holds onto resentments and anger he may hold onto life longer, even when his physical body is ready to cease functioning.

Family and friends, as well as a hospice nurse and social worker may be able to help. They can ask questions of the dying person to understand this frustration and anger, they can listen to the old grievances and issues, and they can suggest ways of putting things in perspective, and letting go of something that doesn't matter anymore. Sometimes writing a letter to acknowledge their forgiveness and mailing to the individual will really help

Many times the object of hate or animosity is no longer living. The source of angst may from been a parent, who mistreated the dying person when they were a child. The release the person feels is not dependent of the presence of the object of their earlier anger. It is just a release of their heart.

Forgiving yourself

Forgiving yourself may be even harder to do than forgiving others. From childhood, we are brought up to judge ourselves, and seeing ourselves lacking, we feel guilty forever. Forgiving yourself requires you first take responsibility and acknowledge to yourself what you really did or said, and then to understand the impact you had on another person. This is a delicate balance. You need to be ruthlessly honest with yourself, while at the same time you need to be compassionate toward yourself. This process can take time if it's a deep and closely guarded guilt. The impetus of dying or having a loved one approaching death can focus the mind intensely and push someone into making this gigantic leap. Dying isn't called the final stage of growth for nothing.

The next step is to acknowledge what you have done and said, to the person involved, and express your sorrow. If the dying person can't say this in person, then he may choose to write a letter and express it. If he is no longer able to do this, he can dictate a letter to someone else. Writing those feelings down, and acknowledging them in a concrete way, really makes a difference. Of course people would love to see a fond reconciliation, a family reunited around a deathbed. This does happen, but it isn't a requirement for the dying person to be able to experience a release from the feeling of guilt.

Reconnections
Forgiving ourselves and forgiving others seem to be a precursor to a complete reconnecting of people who have been estranged for a long time. Many people long for such a connection, even though they haven't done their internal work of forgiving and the other party hadn't done their growth work either. So even if reconciliation is only going to go part of the way, it really helps the dying person put a part of his nagging history behind him.

Hospice people caring for the dying person and his family—the nurse, social worker and spiritual coordinator—know how important it is for everyone's well being to heal some of the traumatic events of the past. They will ask questions about the family so they understand whether anyone is missing from the inner circle, and if so, whether that really is of concern to the patient. Appropriate questions asked of the dying person, as they come close to the end of their lives are, " What is keeping you here? What things do you need to do and say before you are ready to let go and leave?"

Sometimes a family member will make contact with the estranged member, who is often a grown child. They will explain the parent's disease and life expectancy, and ask him to return and visit. Sometimes they come and sometimes the meeting is incredibly healing for the whole family. A dying person may have been able to drop their animosity of previous years, all those issues and reasons don't seem so important any more. If he can love, accept, and give, when the almost stranger arrives, and the visitor is willing to be transformed, the long awaited reunion can be totally joyous. The hospice people involved are also so moved when this happens, that they will often shed tears, too.

If may be that the dying person has gone through such a change in these last years or months that he sees life in a different way. All the details of a long life that seemed so important before don't have much significance in his final days. Love and peace are all that matters now. Many times hospice people talk about visiting wonderful people, who are just a joy to be with, as they have dropped the pretenses of life, and are just who they are, the soul shining through. This event can heal and transform the life of the person who has been estranged. Coming to peace in our heart is the essence of life itself.

Now this is an ideal situation that doesn't always occur. The reluctant child may come home under parental or sibling pressure, but not be able to let go of the old hurts, and the dying person may not be able to let go of his issues. The two people may never have been able to be close. The wounds were too great, for maybe one or both of them, too injured to make a clean switch in attitude. However, being there makes a difference. The survivor will lessen any feelings of guilt and the dying person may find relief in seeing them again. The limited connection was as good as it could have been, and that was a whole lot better than none at all.

Unfortunately in a good many situations the estranged person refuses to come to see the dying person. Perhaps the most heart rendering is when a former spouse prevents children from visiting their other dying parent. The dying person has to come to terms with this in some way. If he can come to peace over it, he will allow himself to die more peacefully. The social worker may suggest he writes a letter to the person they cannot see, expressing all they would like to say. He may just be able to dictate it and have someone write it for him, and then read it back. It doesn't matter if it even ever gets mailed, the act of writing it can be the release and resolution of the emotions involved.

The Family Vigil

The dying process is extremely hard for the dying person. He has to face illness and all its implications, and the fact that he will lose everything, all his things, and all people he has loved. The family, too, has an incredibly difficult task ahead: to care for, nurture, and love someone who really needs their support, while all their emotions cry out with the pain of the loss that will be theirs.

This family vigil comes in as many flavors as there are families. The progression of the disease varies tremendously. One family may have to cope with the slow, slow loss of a loved one to Alzheimer's. This disease takes away the person you knew and loved, little by little, while giving the caretaker an enormous burden of care that lasts for years. Cancer is another word that invokes fear. Cancer may be treated very successfully and go into remission for years. Patient and family still live with not knowing of whether or when it will reoccur. Treatments are hard to endure and may go on a long time. Chronic diseases such as lung or heart problems may leave a patient with severely limited capabilities for a long time. So the nature of the disease varies tremendously and impacts everyone involved.

We think of a family vigil as what happens in a formal sense, when the family gathers around the deathbed, summoned just in time, and then waits for the dying person to leave. It a sudden illness or accident, this may be true. The family gathers for the last few days and stand around the bedside, usually in a hospital.

In a hospice care situation, the dying process may happen over a much longer period of time, as the patient slowly moves toward the end of his life. If the patient is to be cared for at home, it may place different responsibilities on the family. The physical capabilities of the family to care for the patient also vary tremendously. Hospice care in your own home supports the caregiver, so you will also need to explain to them how round the clock care will be provided when it becomes necessary. A loving spouse may be present and capable of being the caregiver. Parents or willing children may also be the primary support. Many dying people are capable of taking care of themselves with almost daily visits from hospice, until quite close to the end. Sometimes people hire round the clock help in the home, or plan on transferring to a nursing home or a hospice residence, or have a family member or friend live with them, when they come close to the end. Hospice support can continue even if the dying person eventually needs to transfer to a care facility home when no one is able to provide care at his home.

The physical care can be enormously draining. The emotional side of the loss is usually the worst aspect. So many families tell us that they were so glad they were able to keep their loved one at home, but they couldn't have done it without hospice. A single caregiver may be overwhelmed taking care of someone 24 hours a day 7 days a week, so they do need to ask for help and relief from other family members, friends, hospice volunteers, and paid care takers. Hospice benefit also provides care by funding the dying person's placement in a care facility for a few days to provide a needed respite.

I have often expressed my awe of caregivers of the dying, in my bereavement groups. My personal experience was in vigil with dying family members for short periods, and as a hospice volunteer where I just spent a few hours with the dying person. I have often said, that I don't think I would be that good, and I get quite unpleasant when I'm sleep deprived. Each caregiver replied, that he never expected he would be able to do it, but when the situation arose, he just did what needed to be done.

The nature of the relationship

The emotional load experienced by the people around the dying person depends on the nature of their relationship. This is pretty obvious at one level—usually watching spouses dying is harder than watching parents dying; watching young people dying is harder than watching old people dying. But at another level the depth of our connection with someone can vary enormously, even if the relationship is defined in the same way.

One older lady told me of the devastating impact of her husband's death 20 years earlier. She didn't know how to drive and yet lived remotely, and she didn't know how to write a check as her husband had taken care of all that kind of thing. So she faced not only the shock of losing her life partner, but also her own ability to cope in the world.

Another lady in her 60's was equally devastated by her husband's death, because she had no one else in the world to which she could turn. She was capable of handling her own financial affairs to a certain extent, and could manage on a practical level, but this one person had met all her social needs. They had shared a view that you couldn't trust anyone outside the two of them, so after he died she was incredibly lonely. She did accept hospice personnel as people she could trust and as people who would accept her, so she welcomed my visits.

An offspring had stayed home and lived with her mother all her life. She was there to take care of her mother as she aged and finally died, but the one key relationship in her life was this parent so she, too, became totally lost at her mother's death. One man said that he and his mother was a couple, in the sense that they were together all day, every day, and shared all details of everyday living.

So one of the concerns the hospice people will have is about the stability of the family after the death. They may encourage the dying person to do what he can that will help his family later. This will include writing a will, putting things in order, teaching loved ones how to do the things that they will be called upon to do for themselves in the future. This vigil, standing together in the unfolding process, is a two way street.

Emotional maturity

I was able to handle the death my mother in a very different way, from how I had handled the death of my father, 10 years earlier. I had a closer bond to my mother, and you might have thought I would have had a much harder time. The difference was the 10 years that had passed in time, and in my own growth. I had faced my own fear of death, come to understand my own separateness and connectedness. So with my mother, I was very clear I was there to support her, and help her die peacefully. Now when I am faced with loss, I will cry and feel all my feelings intensely, but I know who I am in the world, and I know I will cope.

Anticipatory grief

People experience grief in their own way. As we cannot

know what someone else is feeling, we have to accept his form of grief, and validate his process. When a man knows his loved one will die he will deal with it in his own way. Some people will accept it as reality, but make the most of each day, while others will deny it to the final day. Some loved ones begin to grieve ahead of time, and then can be concerned later, when they judge themselves as not grieving enough after the funeral.

I know I cried and cried the day my father told me that he had lung cancer, because I knew this was going to end his life. I had worked with lung cancer patients before, and knew the outlook, given that he was nearly 80 years old. He lived another 18 months, and I didn't cry much at the time of his death, because I had done my grieving earlier.

I led a support group one day and 2 women each talked of taking care of her dying husband for 10 years. One said, "Well I was getting used to it over the 10 years, knowing he was dying, so I am beginning to adjust now, and the other woman said, " Well, I didn't expect him to die, it was a complete shock when it happened." During the progression of the disease, it was clear to everyone else that the disease was terminal, but she had never been able to accept it.

Each person grieves in his own way and at his own pace, but if he grieves ahead of the death, he may adjust faster to the lost after the death. One woman shared her fear that she wasn't grieving enough after her husband's death, but felt relieved when I pointed out how much grief has had expressed before he actually died.

Being with the dying
The emphasis here is on being. Visitors who come to visit with the intent of being a cheerleader, of convincing you need more resolve to live, or just to avoid the reality by talking about

the inconsequential, aren't much use, and are definitely exhausting.

A friend with lung cancer told me of her long time friend, who rushed up to her, hugged her, and cried and cried. My friend just stood there, but said to me later, "Why did she expect me to comfort *her*? I don't need to deal with *her* distress and loss. I have enough of my own."

In training hospice volunteers to be with the dying, we focus on having them listen, being still, and having them pick up their cues from the dying person. We need to put aside all our own issues, check them at the door to reclaim later. All that is required is that we walk in to the patient's home with a warm heart, happy to be there, in whatever way suits the dying person that day. It also includes sitting quietly, reading a book, ready to help if needed, but not a visitor who requires entertaining.

Sometimes a hospice patient does want us to talk about things outside his room. If he is bored with his restricted view of the world, someone who brings sunshine into the house can be very welcome. I visited one wonderful lady, who was restricted to wheel chair and bed, but she had been an avid gardener, so each week I would take one flower of each plant flowering in my garden, and we would go through them one by one. She would tell me the Latin name, whether she had grown it before, and the best way to take care of them. Different volunteers can offer different things. Some give a brief massage, some will bring books or music, or play an instrument, but following what ever lead the dying person has given. Sometimes, bringing a beloved pet into a resident care facility is a comfort.

What do the dying want from us?

Dame Saunders wrote, "I once asked a man who was dying

what he needed above all in those who were caring for him. He said, 'For someone to look as if they are trying to understand me'. Indeed, it is impossible to understand fully another person, but I never forgot that he did not ask for success, but only that someone should care enough to try." *8

Dying people want what we all want, to be loved and accepted. They may appreciate being touched, as many people pull away at their appearance. Many times in the course of my work with hospice, I have been thanked for caring. It seems such a small thing to offer. I care, but it seems to make a huge difference.

Dying people also liked to be valued for their lifetime of knowledge and experience. I used to visit another lady who had been an expert in quilting, and still tried to continue these efforts, although her eyesight was failing. I bought myself some fabric to take with me each week, so that she could be my teacher, and we would sit together sewing as we talked.

Compassion

Stephen Levine said, "When your fear touches someone's pain it becomes pity, when your love touches someone's pain it becomes compassion."*9 This is so true. We can't really be there for someone, and be her companion until we let go of our own fear, or at least are willing to let the dying person be our teacher.

Ideally we need to show a dying person unconditional love. How do we do that? Sogyal Rinpoche writes of practices to help us develop compassion in his book, The Tibetan Book of Living and Dying.

I think that dying people have taught me compassion, even though I don't quite understand how that happened. I was fearful when I went to my first dying patient, mostly because I was scared he might need medical or physical help that I was unable to give. I felt an incredible love when I was with him, a love that came for him, that flowed through me, or through him, I couldn't figure out which it was. I didn't understand it at all. I am far from unique. Thousand of people who work with the dying would say the same thing. I would also find myself giving a patient a hug or a kiss, and I didn't understand that either. I saw them beautiful in some way, which belied their physical appearance.

Fear does mask these feelings. It is much easier to be a volunteer who walks into a family, knowing this person will die soon, than to be caregiver who has to face losing his loved one, and a part of himself. Fear is bound to be a big component, when you are in the situation that is affecting all your present and your future.

Coming close to the end of life

The family and hospice will do everything in their power to make the comfort of the dying person paramount. Support for changing physical symptoms will be adjusted as soon as necessary, and the family will know what to do, and how to react, to some "what if" scenarios. All things possible will be done to keep the person dying as comfortable as possible, and to support the family.

The family and hospice will also have done everything they can possibly do to help the person be ready mentally, emotionally, and spiritually. The greatest gift loved ones can offer is to tell their loved one that they will be able to cope without him, although they will miss him terribly, and will always remember him; then tell him that he can leave when he needs to. If they can say this, and really mean it, the dying person will feel free to leave, when they are ready. The atmosphere needs to be calm and quiet. Touching, holding, climbing in bed with to hold the dying person is appropriate if desired. Even so, when many loved ones expect to be present, and not let them die alone, the person actually dies when a loved one is outside the room. Perhaps it was just too hard to leave their loved one if they were in the room.

Specific Spiritual Needs

In dying, people need spiritual support, in a way that helps them. This is not the time to try to change anyone's beliefs. They may have been devout follower in a particular religion, or may decide to return to beliefs of their childhood. The priest, minister, rabbi, pastor or whatever else their spiritual support may be named, will be called in, or the hospice spiritual coordinator or chaplain will be available to anyone who chooses to accept it. Many people without any specific religion, may be comforted by their own belief in an afterlife, and may want to express their own thoughts and feelings.

To die peacefully the person has to be ready to let go of their attachments to this life: places, things, and people. Sogyal Rinpoche says, "The last thought or emotion that we have before we die has an extremely powerful determining effect on our immediate future." [10] The Buddhist may have concerns about the kind of life they will be reborn into, but Christians also have concerns about their immediate future. So a peaceful loving environment supports all people and all beliefs.

After death occurs

After death occurs, a survivor may hold to the body of their loved one for a long time, literally holding on, not wanting to accept the death as reality. Some people sit and cry, some people wander off to other parts of the house, not able to believe that death has occurred. There is a whole range of responses.

If the person has died at home, under hospice care, and the nurse isn't already present, the first task would be to call hospice. The nurse will come to be with the family and usually to formally pronounce the death. She will gently wash the body, and the caregiver can help her if she chooses to. The social worker will also come to the home if there are particular concerns about how a loved one is likely to react.

No matter how well prepared the family is, death itself is still a shock.

Signs of the Death Process

If the dying person and her loved ones have made the decision to stay in her own home, and use the services of a hospice for in-home care, then the caretaker needs to understand what can be expected as that person nears the end of his life. Caring for a dying person at home, is one of the most difficult tasks that anyone has to face Fear of the unknown is relieved a little by information, which will prepare the caretaker for what may transpire. Knowing that he can call the hospice nurse at any time is also very comforting.

Knowing what to expect, and how to respond, will give everyone a shared feeling of support, understanding, and comfort. Being honest and as straightforward as possible with each other enables the family to face their fears.

In general, though, two processes proceed at the same time. There are physical signs and symptoms of approaching death, as well as emotional, spiritual, and mental signs. Understanding them helps the caregivers respond appropriately. Each person is unique and will react in their own way, and not all signs and symptoms occur in every person, or in the same order. The two processes are closely interrelated and interdependent.

Physical Signs
When the dying person enters the final stage before death, the body begins the final phase of shutting down. This process ends when all the body's organs stop working and death occurs. Usually this process happens in an orderly and progressive series of physical changes, which are expected, and are the body's way of preparing itself to stop. These changes are not medical emergencies and do not require intervention, except for checking the dying person is comfortable.

The hospice nurse will have a good idea, especially after consulting with the medical director, of the possible turns and effects this particular disease will have. She will be watching out for changes on her regular visits, and she will warn the family what is likely to happen, and what could possible happen, as the disease progresses. She will also be able to have the family prepared for how they will cope, including having the right medications in the house, so they wouldn't have to wait for new doctors orders, and medication delivery.

The focus will be on keeping the dying person as comfortable as possible, and pain free. Initially the person may be quite mobile, but as his mobility decreases, aids, such as walkers, a hospital bed, commode, transfer mechanism from bed to commode, perhaps a catheter, will be introduced to support him. Again the hospice personnel will make suggestions and recommendations, but leave the dying person to make the choice.

As the body gradually shuts down the person will lose his appetite. Accepting this as normal may be hard for the caretaker, because nurturing and caring for someone is often associated with eating well. The appetite may fall off gradually, although the person may still enjoy special treats. As long as it does no harm, treats are a good way to lift the spirits. As he comes closer to death, the need for liquids gradually decreases. The demand on the body, to process intravenous fluids, is not helpful. The dying person will appreciate having their mouth moistened so it doesn't become too dry, perhaps with crushed ice or juice chips or just with a small sponge applicator. Naturally as the body takes in less and less fluid the urine becomes concentrated and may become tea colored. It can also reduce because of a decrease in circulation through the kidneys. The dying person may become incontinent.

The person may spend more and more time sleeping and be more difficult to arouse or unresponsive. This is normal change is due in part to changes in the metabolism of the body. The dying person can appreciate the quiet companion who doesn't need to talk much, but is there, maybe holding his hand. Speak to the person as you normally would, and don't talk about them to others in the room. Hearing is the last of the senses to be lost.

The body's ability to maintain a constant temperature weakens so the person's hands and arms, legs and feet may feel increasingly cold to the touch. The color of the skin may change, with the underside of his body becoming darker and the skin may be mottled. This is just sign that the circulation of blood is slowing down to the body's extremities and is being reserved for the more essential organs. The person just needs to be kept warm with a blanket.

Sometimes the person becomes disoriented and may be confused about the identity of people, the time, the place. It helps if the caretakers identify themselves gently, communicating clearly and simply. The dying person may make restless and repetitive motions such as pulling at bed linen or clothing. This can be due to less blood getting to the brain. Speaking in a calm natural way may be all that is needed to calm the person down.

The breathing pattern becomes slower and more erratic. Close to the end, breathing can stop for as much as forty five seconds before resuming again. Congestion can also be very loud. Oral secretions may increase and collect in the back of the throat. This is sometimes referred to as the death rattle.

Emotional, spiritual and mental signs

When the person's body is ready and wanting to stop, but the person has some important issue or relationship that is unresolved or not yet reconciled, they may tend to linger even if they are uncomfortable or debilitated, in order to finish whatever needs finishing. On the other hand, when a person is emotionally, spiritually and mentally resolved and ready for release, but his body had not completed its final physical process, the person will continue to live until the physical shut down is completed.

As the dying person prepares to release himself from this life he completes his business with some people, effectively saying goodbye, and focusing on a smaller group of close family or even just one person, and spending more and more time withdrawn. This appearance of an unresponsive, or comatose state is a preparation for a release from surroundings and relationships. Sometimes the caregiver needs to protect the dying person from too many visitors and respectfully ask them to say their goodbyes quietly and leave.

Restless behavior can be a physical sign or an emotional one indicating that something is still unresolved or unfinished. The hospice nurse or social worker will help the caretaker try to identify any issues that may be holding the person here, and try to find ways of releasing them from tension or fear.

Again, the greatest gift the immediate family can give to the dying person is permission to die and leave them. A dying person may hold onto life as long as possible, even though the body is ready to leave, because he are so concerned that his loved one cannot cope without him. The family needs to say everything that completes their life with the dying person, including, "I love you" and "Goodbye," which aids his peaceful passing enormously.

The dying person may also have vision like experiences or unusual dreams in the last week or two. They may claim to have seen or spoken to people who are already dead, or seen places not presently accessible to others. The surrounding family may see and hear the dying person, listen to something they alone can hear or speaking to people they alone can see. These experiences are very real to the dying person, and quite normal and common. The caregiver can just accept them as real, even if she can't confirm their presence. The dying person might need reassurance that these experiences are normal. This is very common in the last week or two before death. It would appear that loved ones who have already died, come back with the purpose of accompanying the dying person over from this life.

Close to the end the person may make statements that seem to come from out of the blue. This indicates he is ready to say goodbye and is testing whether the loved one is ready to say goodbye, too.

Timing
Everyone is unique, so all these symptoms will not occur in all people, and the timing of events can vary dramatically. In

sudden death there is no warning, events have a life of their own. Some people may have only hours or a few days, from knowing the severity of their illness to their death. Some people may be dying over a ten-year period. As a person reconciles the issues and relationships of a lifetime, he seems more able to release himself from this world peacefully.

Some dying people seem to know ahead of time when they will die, and some seem to be able to choose the best moment to do so.

Death

The experience we call death occurs when the body completes the natural process of both physically shutting down, and completing the emotional, spiritual, and mental aspects. These two processes need to happen in a way, that is appropriate and unique to the values, beliefs and life style of the dying person.

The signs of death are: no breathing, no heartbeat, loss of bowel and bladder control, no response to shaking or shouting, eyelids slightly open, eyes fixed on a certain spot, and jaw relaxed and mouth slightly open.

Signs of spirit

Sometimes a survivor describes the body of his loved one some time later, maybe within an hour of his death, and say it looked totally different, that it was clear that the essence of the person was no longer there. Some people describe seeing some matter or essence leave the body at the moment breathing ceases or shortly thereafter.

A dying person may struggle in their process, and then suddenly come to peace a few days before she dies. Often people, who come to this place of peace, are described as having a look of wonder, a beautiful smile, as if they have seen what is to come and are very happy about it. Some dying people seem to glow from within for the last days or even weeks.

Many witnesses of a dying person observe light and energy around the person, and feel a difference in the level of love surrounding them. Some people describe the dying person as the source of that love and sometimes, they describe beings of light in attendance around the person dying. I certainly saw beings of light around my mother as she was dying.

This is life's final mystery.

The Act of Dying: Slipping from This World into the Next

But is the while I think on thee, dear friend. All the losses are restored and sorrow's end.
—Shakespeare

The end
In hospice staff meetings, a nurse will say, "It's not going to be long now, she is already talking to her dead mother." It is very common for someone coming close to death, which might just a week or so away, to see people no one else sees. It's as if their dead family and friends come to collect them to take them over the other side. The patient may say, "I'm not ready to go yet." Sometimes the patient has an exceptionally vivid dream, so vivid he might describe it as real, of being somewhere else.

One foot in either world
Sometimes the patient might be the translator between this

world and the next, as he stands with one foot in either camp. Like John for example:

John

I visited a delightful hospice patient in a nursing home. His wife would spend the day at his bedside but didn't want him to be alone in the evening when she returned to her home. So I, as a hospice volunteer, went to sit beside him. After many visits I loved being with John. He was kind hearted and caring, a very special man.

One day it was clear he was getting close to the end, much of his time was spent in a semi coma. I just stood by the bed, watching him. He would become conscious, open his eyes and try to say something. I could tell what he wanted to say was very important, and I would lean closer. On one occasion he said: "Love is all!" I repeated it and he just beamed at me, so pleased that I had understood. He slept again, and awoke a second time. He tried to communicate again, and I repeated what I thought he had said in order to be absolutely clear. "It's all in the eyeball." Again he was happy I had it right.

I went into work the next day and wrote those words in large letters and pinned them on my wall. What truths to live by! Love is all that matters, and maybe that is all we will meet when we leave this life. Then, too, so much depends on our way of seeing and on what we expect to see. If we expect to find threatening people we will; if we expect to find loving, supportive people, then we will. It is all in the eyeball.

Frank

Another elderly man, Frank, was dying at home under hospice care. His large family knew he was coming close to the end of his life and they gathered around his bed. The time of Frank's dying had been a time for the family to put aside many of their differences; an estranged child had returned to the family fold. They had worked through many of the issues that had held them apart for years, and Frank and his family were at peace.

Frank was lying in his bed propped by many pillows and talked to his family. The conversation was much more than they had expected. Frank spoke to his son and his daughter-in-law who had lost a child, John, in a car crash, he said, " John wants you to know he is just fine." To his wife he said, "Your mother is fine and says she likes the new outfit you just bought." Her mother had died 30 years earlier. Frank went around the room making comments to each person from someone they knew who had died.

Frank seemed to stand with one foot in this world and one foot in the next. He was able to be the communicator between those worlds, and provide answers to the questions he knew people in his family had lived with for a long time.

People very close to death seem to be partly in this world and partly in another. They might see and hear things we can't hear; they may know things about other people who have been long gone. They may come to greater understanding of what their lives have been about. Books such as "Life after Life" by Raymond Moody, document experiences people have had who were clinically dead and then come back. Naturally we don't have recorded experiences of people who don't return, except through channeling, so it is impossible for me to expand or be absolute in this regard. Perhaps he tunnel the dying see with a light at the end, is the experience only of those who are to come back.

Timing

Frequently the dying person seems to be able to time his death. Some people live on and frequently continue to suffer. They give their family more time to make the adjustments required. They need to know the people they love will cope if they die. It is a real gift if the loved ones can say from their heart, "I will be all right. I will miss you, but it is okay if you die now." Then the patient is free.

William

Claire's father had undergone some severe debilitating tests 10 months prior to his death. The doctor had indicated that he would die quite soon after the tests. The family was outraged about what they perceived to be poor medical treatment and were quite determined that their relative, husband and father would live longer than the medical profession predicted and have some good quality time before he died.

William survived against the odds and lived for 10 months. Finally the family accepted the doctor's prognosis that there was nothing more that they could be done to cure him and arranged his transfer from hospital to a hospice care live-in facility. Within 15 minutes of his arrival at the hospice facility, Claire's father died.

This man was able to rally around, even though the doctors thought he was dying because that was clearly what his family wanted. When he was moved to the hospice he knew the family had accepted the fact he was dying and he knew he no longer needed to struggle to live on for them so he was able to let go quickly and die peacefully.

Chuck

The hospice nurse had warned the family a day or so in advance that Gary's father was close to dying. Each person in the house had his chance to say final words to him in the knowledge that he was hearing them. Gary had called his twenty year-old son, who was at work and advised him that now was the time to come to his grandfather's bedside. Gary told his father to hang on until his grandson arrived.

The hospice nurse, who was sitting on the bed holding the old man, said, "Your father may prefer to die before his grandson arrives so he spares him the pain of watching him go." Within minutes, as Gary and the nurse were lifting him back onto his pillows, he made a strange noise as the last breath released from his lungs, and died.

Gary did say he felt something leave his father's body and then the body looked so different. It didn't look like his father anymore.

This was the man who had been able to hold onto life so long for the sake of the people he loved. He wanted to know they were going to be all right without him. He was even able to choose the moment of his death in order not to disturb his grandson.

Sometimes the patient seems to know exactly when they will die, but no one else can understand what they are talking about. One nurse who worked in a nursing home shared the following story with me.

"This old man in my ward told me in late summer that November 15th was a very important day. Weeks later he mentioned it again and asked whether I would be around that day. More weeks went by and he brought up the subject again. I thought is was no more than the rambling mind of an old man, but yes, he died on November 15th."

Patient visions

A hospice chaplain told me of a dying man she had visited. She and the hospice nurse were sitting either side of his bed, because they believed the man's death was imminent. He had been quite weak for six weeks or more, he was unable to sit up unaided.

The chaplain decided to sing a hymn that she knew he liked. After a few minutes the dying man sat bolt upright and said, "I saw angels! I saw angels! And they were singing so beautifully."

The man died with a smile on his face just a short time afterward.

When dreams presage death

Elizabeth

Elizabeth told me of her dream that presaged the death of her mother-in-law. Always her mother-in-law had been critical and disapproving of Elizabeth. Elizabeth had divorced her son twelve years prior to this dream and Elizabeth had had no contact with her ex-mother-in-law. This is the dream.

"My mother-in-law was standing on the stairs, holding onto the ornate Victorian stair rail and looked down on her family gathered in the hall below. She read through a list of all that was wrong with her. I thought that was very odd because she never complained in her life."

The following morning Elizabeth's daughter called her. She told her that her mother-in-law had died the night before. Elizabeth tried to understand why she would be the one to have the dream, and concluded she was the only one who would be willing to give her mother-in-law permission to die and would not be holding on to her to stay alive

Taffy

I had a dog, which at the age of eleven years old, had a number of aliments, but seemed to be doing well. My previous dog had lived to thirteen, so I guess I expected this dog to live another couple of years.

One night I had a very clear dream in which I understood that my dog was dying. The dog came to me in the dream still looking quite healthy, but I knew she would die soon.

When I awoke I knew that the dream was to give me warning that this dog would die, so the dream gave me time to grow accustomed to the idea.

A couple of months later, I took Taffy to the vets to put her to sleep rather than let her suffer. She had internal cancer masses and could no longer digest any food. With animals, I find that final drive to the vets incredibly sad, but I always felt my dogs told me at some point that they had suffered enough, so I didn't doubt I was doing the right thing.

Knowing Taffy would be comforted by my presence and with tears streaming down my face, I agreed to hold my pet while the vet administered the fatal shot.

The vet monitored the heartbeat and then told me it had stopped and the dog was dead. For one crazy minute I wondered whether this was reversible. Then I remembered I didn't want Taffy to suffer. It was clear to me that Taffy still looked like Taffy, and that the spirit of Taffy was still in that body. The vet said she would leave me alone with the body for a few minutes. In my mind I talked to Taffy, explaining to her that her body was worn out now and she was free to leave. I was aware of the spirit leaving the body and hanging about 3 feet above her head. I looked down and saw the body, it was nothing but a pile of skin and bones, a body that was clearly no longer occupied.

A few months after Taffy's death, I had a beautiful dream where I was in the garden on a beautiful day and Taffy came running to me. Both of us were overjoyed to see each other. My grief was over after that warm experience.

Sensations

Martha's mother

Martha had taken care of her mother during three years of illness. For the last four months her mother was receiving care from hospice, and Martha was able to continue to be her caretaker with that support. Eventually the hospice nurse warned Martha that her mother was likely to die within a day or so.

Martha's mother became weaker and weaker and was confined to bed. Martha sat next to her on the bed, but, as her breath became more labored, she was suddenly aware that "her mother" was floating up near the ceiling and looking down on her body.

When I questioned Martha more closely, she said even though she was looking at her mother's lifeless body on the bed, she was totally convinced she could sense the presence of her mother's energy floating out of the body.

Peace

Many people seem to come to a very peaceful state a day or two before they die, and then they slip away quietly.

Susan

I was invited to join a group of women, who met monthly in order to give one another support. I already knew four members of their group of six. I had not met Susan, but had heard about her frequently from these women and another common friend.

She had been fighting cancer for several years and no longer seemed to be responding to treatment. We sat around a circular table in a restaurant and shared our stories, our hopes and fears.

Susan talked about what was happening to her. She cried and asked for our support as she confessed how frightened she was. Having exhausted all other medical options, she was planning a trip to Mexico for a miracle cure. Despite the fact that I knew she would not live long, we planned our next monthly meeting around Susan's availability. I hugged her, said goodbye and offered my energetic help.

After a couple of weeks I found Susan was much in my thoughts. I talked to mutual friends and learned she was going downhill fast. I kept meditating, praying, and focusing my mind on her. One Friday night, as I was driving home I felt her ask for my help in leaving her body. I summoned all the energy I could (given the need to drive safely) to help her lift off. I thought I hadn't been able to help enough. I wasn't sure she had moved over. I checked the time on the car clock; it was 6 p.m. During the weekend I sensed her at peace, surrounded by love.

Finally I heard that Susan died on Monday after that weekend, furthermore her closest friend who was with her told me that on the Friday at 6 p.m. she had seen something in the nature of a beatific vision and became totally at peace until she died three days later. The family and friends who surrounded Susan in those last few days, felt sure Susan was moving on to something quite wonderful. The sense of peace and love encompassed her, clearly she felt sustained by it.

We do seem to be connected to each other in ways we can't explain. Many people tell of an event that occurred at the exact time of death. Often they talk of just knowing what had happened.

Many people have described an incredible sense of peace

and love, which fill the room in the last few days. For each of them the experience has been unique.

Death: the actual moment

A nurse who had been on duty in an emergency room told me a story about the separation of spirit and body.

After a severe car crash a man struggled to maintain his hold on life. His distraught family surrounded him: they were in shock and not prepared to let him go. He held on to life until his family left the room and then he quietly slipped away. The nurse said she had seen this happen many times. Someone would hold on because that's what their family wanted them to do, only when they were on their own, would they die quietly.

Hospice nurses have commented on the numerous occasions that they have watch people will die in the absence of the family. They seem to choose not to go when loved ones are there. Perhaps it is too hard to leave or maybe they wish to spare their nearest and dearest some grief. People seem to be able to choose the time when they die.

A hospice nurse described another family gathering:

A dying woman was very close to the end, after each having spoken and said goodbye, her husband, three of her four children, her brother and sister surrounded the bed. The woman held on and held on until her second child, her son, Steve, came into the room and stood at her bedside. His mother looked at him and said, "Steve, I love you," and smiled. Then she took her last breath, and died.

Time and again, patients seem to have had some control over when they died. They hold on because someone needs them to do so or because they want to see something or someone. When they have finished their business and said goodbye they are able to let go peacefully.

Judith

The most striking telepathic experience I ever had was with a hospice patient named Judith. I had been visiting her on Tuesday evenings each week for a few months. Initially, if you were right there for her to lean on, she could walk. She would move from the sofa to the veranda for a smoke and could go to the bathroom or to the kitchen. As time passed she became more and more frail. I would help her a sofa to a wheelchair, to the bathroom, and finally from hospital bed to a commode. She would talk about her life, and share her pain at what was happening to her. She was a wonderful lady, very caring, and very concerned about leaving her family and the impact her death would have on them. I respected her highly and loved her. I knew her end was approaching.

One Thursday at work, I was in a rather boring all day meeting, so I let myself daydream about Judith, in the knowledge that she was close to death, I was thinking about how I might be able to help her on my next visit on the following Tuesday,. I pictured myself by her bed, channeling light to her with my hands. She was in my thoughts frequently for the next 24 hours.

The next morning as I took my place at the same conference table in a continuation of the same boring meeting, I instantly found myself, at least in the picture in my mind, standing behind Judith and we both took off out of the tops of our heads. We went up and up together very quickly. When I looked up I saw light beings waiting for her. I knew they were there to receive Judith to the other side. Judith continued on to meet them and I immediately came back to my body, content with knowing that she was with loved ones, and rejoined my meeting.

I thought that was an interesting daydream, until I got home that evening. Hospice personnel had left a message on my answering machine to say that Judith had died that morning.

Who knows what is reality or whose reality we are talking about? Much later I read Isabel Allende's book, *Paula*, the story of her dying daughter. Isobel's experience as her daughter finally died was similar to mine. Perhaps it wasn't all in my imagination?

Many people talk about how different the body looks after someone has died. I feel the same when I view a body at a funeral or a wake. Clearly the body is the preserved outer shell and the spirit of the person is no longer there. For me the presence of the body is superfluous; clearly it is not the person I knew. However, viewing the body does allow one to grasp the fact that the person has gone.

Through her own tears, a daughter of another hospice patient told me the story of her mother's dying:

"She just slipped away so peacefully with a beautiful smile on her face. Even though she was no longer breathing I could tell her spirit was still there and her face was still smiling. I didn't notice the actual moment she left her body, but certainly within an hour she was gone, and all that was left was this empty shell with no smile. That shell was not my mother."

The difference between a body occupied by "life" or "soul" is totally different from the empty shell of a body. Many of the bereaved describe the body of their loved one in the same way. Some see the shift quickly, and some say an hour later it looked very different. This may be wishful thinking or a physiological effect, but clearly it is a healing process for the bereaved.

A hospital nurse described the death of a patient that she witnessed. A terminally ill patient was assigned to a free room in the post surgical ward that this nurse worked on. The dying woman had been at home, but was admitted to hospital when her family could no longer manage her care. The family had spent the day at her bedside, and as evening was approaching, they left to return home. The nurse stopped by the room after the last person left, to check that the patient was comfortable.

The lights were dim; the atmosphere felt very calm and very quiet, after the turbulent presence of the family. The nurse knew that the patient didn't have long to live. She pulled up a chair next to the bed and held the dying woman's hand. After 5 minutes or so, the patient took a few slow deep breaths about a minute apart. After a minute or so after her last breath, the nurse looked up and saw that the room was spinning, she saw it go faster and faster like a tornado. She felt both excited and scared. The "tornado" touched down, and the nurse, still holding the patient's hand, felt that the patient had gone and the body in the bed was an empty shell. She described that she felt dizzy herself. Within moments a nursing assistant came in and said, "Did she die?" The nurse did the after care of the body very gently and tenderly, and said she felt she didn't feel bad about that death because she knew the right thing had happened.

Sudden death

Sometimes the whole process of dying is dramatically shortened, and a loved one dies very quickly from an accident or from a massive coronary. Survivors will rationalize the death and say how much better it was for the deceased because they didn't have to suffer. It can be doubly difficult for the bereaved, though; they had no time, as would have been possible during a protracted illness, to come to accept that their loved one was dying.

John

Miriam's husband suffered a massive heart attack. She was

with him the whole time from the onset of the initial symptoms to his death, which occurred within a few hours. She said, "We were lying in bed and at 4.30 in the morning, John woke up concerned about a business deal and explained to me what he had decided to do. I must have dozed off again, because at 5 am I was awakened by this horrible noise. He was no longer beside me in the bed, but sitting bolt upright in the bedroom chair. His eyes were vacant and he was this ash gray color. I just knew he was halfway gone. At that moment my heart and mind were one; I called the ambulance and then tried to lower him to the floor. I was aware of every nuance in that short time before the EMTs arrived. John's energy was above me; I could feel him watching me, and my every move. I went with him in the ambulance and sat in the waiting room while the hospital staff did everything they could. Still, I could feel John hovering over me, with love and concern. I was aware I was trying to explain away the feeling, maybe it's because I'm hyperventilating. It was a profound, poignant and clear experience.

At 7 a.m. the doctor came to tell me it was over, John was dead. I went into to see his body, but I didn't like to be there at all. It wasn't John. The very essence of what he was had left. No longer did I feel his energy with me."

Had John lived perhaps he would have described an out of body experience, he might have described watching his wife throughout her time of terror and anxiety. John's energy had certainly stayed with his wife through that intensely difficult experience.

Summary
So many of these stories have a common thread. The patients are preparing to leave this life by completing life's business with the people who are essential to them. When their

business is complete and they are ready to go, they come to a profound place of peace and love, which can be experienced by healthy onlookers. When ready, they do seem to be able to choose the exact moment they leave this world.

Many people talk about the difference between a body with a soul in it, and a body after the soul has left. It is clear that the energy, which made the person alive, has left the body. The body without the presence of that energy or "soul" just isn't that person any more.

Some stories tell of the passage of that energy or soul out of the body.

Family and Friends Bereft

A Native American Prayer:

Do not stand at my grave and weep.
I am not there. I do not sleep.
I am a thousand winds that blow.
I am the diamond glint on snow
I am the sunlight on ripened grain.
I am the gentle Autumn rain.
When you wake in the morning hush.
I am the swift, uplifting rush
Of quiet birds in circling flight.
I am the soft starlight at night.
Do not stand at my grave and weep.
I am not there. I do not sleep.

Their Feelings and Experiences in the Early Days

Shock

Often when the death happens the survivors are in shock. In the early days of loss, the bereaved may hardly feel anything. Numb, with their minds barely aware, their body goes through routines. They may just keep saying they just can't believe this has happened. Even when the loved ones have known someone was dying for years, the actuality sends them into trauma. They cannot believe that death finally occurred. A widow may go through the whole process of organizing a funeral and catering for the company, but remember little of this afterward. They have worked on autopilot, gone through the motions in a state of shock.

Family and friends think the bereaved are coping well. It is not usual for the people who are gathered at the wake or funeral to leave in the belief that the bereaved are handling the death competently or even pretty well indeed. In most instances the truth is quite the contrary. The bereaved have yet to experience the reality of the death of their loved one; the bombshell hasn't yet hit them. It is some time later, when the actuality hits home, that they need support in earnest.

There is nothing wrong with being in a state of shock. This is the way we protect ourselves from having to deal with painful things when we are not up to coping.

Grieving is a process we seem to need to go through in our own timeframe. This first stage of shock and numbness takes as long as it takes, and the work of the bereaved during this stage is to understand the person is dead and won't come back. Some people seem to move through this in hours, and some take years.

People vary in their feelings and how they react. Some people may cry a lot and some cry not at all. Some prefer to do their grieving in some other way. Many get involved in a physical project, such as building a stonewall, where they have to lift heavy boulders. There are as many ways to grieve as there are people grieving.

Naturally there is going to be a major difference between grieving over the loss of a constant, close companion from the sorrow felt for a friend seen once a week or an acquaintance seen on rare occasions. Age is another factor. However devastating the loss of a partner to individuals in their twenties, eventually they are likely to recreate a satisfactory life for themselves, though, of course, they can never replace that loved one. Older widows may have been dependent on their husband for things and have a very hard time in coping with life by themselves. There is a loss of a person, and a loss of the part of the self that was in the relationship with the deceased. Most relationships have good sides and not such good sides, so losses include what was and what might have been.

Most people are still in shock during the first week. Those people who are trying to support the bereaved need to be there and see what support the bereaved need. Usually they need people who are willing to talk and listen. They don't need those well-meaning souls who hand out advice or discourage an expression of grief.

Events that presage the death

Some people have described experiences that occur just as the death occurs. Rarely do they know how to interpret these experiences, but they take on a whole new significance for them once they know about the death and can figure out that the two events happened simultaneously. Some people experience such events and know the significance: their loved one has died.

Phyllis

A good friend had two sets of experiences with telephones. When her mother was dying she was anticipating a phone call in the night to tell her news of her mother's death.

The phone did ring; it rang for three consecutive days. On the first and second occasion Phyllis picked up the receiver, but there was no one there, and when Phyllis went to answer it there was no one there. On the third day she got the message that her mother had died.

A few years later Phyllis' best friend died after a protracted illness that had left her effectively imprisoned in her body. The phone rang again in the middle of the night for several days, and once she heard her friend's voice say "Help me."

Phyllis was convinced the phone calls were a attempts on the part of her mother and dying friend to contact her when they were no longer able to do it physically. Those words "Help me" were extremely distressing for Phyllis to hear.

Dreams

Sometimes the information has come in a dream. The following occurrences exemplify how this can be so.

I learned my father was dead from a dream. My father's cancer had been progressing and he was going downhill steadily. I had visited him and my mother in England a couple of times in the last few months of his life and knew it was just going to be a matter of time before I got the telephone call telling me that he had died. I sleep heavily and normally nothing awakens me in the night. The dream was as follows:

I dreamed my mother was shaking me, trying to wake me up. I dreamed that I woke up and looked at her and she said: "Your father is dead."

When I woke. I knew the dream had been real. I got up and checked the clock; it was just 4 a.m., but I called my mother in England. It was true, my father had died and she had been thinking of me and trying to figure out the right time to call me.

Birds

Often birds are reported to be the go between and information carrier. My brother awoke that same morning of our father's death to the sound of bird song outside his window; in that instant he knew his father had died.

Another couple Barbara and Sam, were awakened during the night by a bird beating its wing against the window. It was very dark still, just 3 am by their alarm clock, not a normal time for birds, other than nocturnal ones, to be about, let alone to be beating its wings on the window pane. Later that morning Barbara and Sam got a phone call to say that the Sam's father had died at 3 a.m.

Weather

Some people can correlate a sudden gust of wind with the time of their loved ones death.

My own experience with that was after I had returned to this country, having left my dying Mother in a hospital in England. I had flown back on the Saturday after the doctors told me it could be three weeks or so until she died. On the Sunday evening I talked to my brother who had been to visit my mother, he thought she was fading fast.

During the night a sudden wind blew and a screen clattered from my bedroom window to the floor. I woke with a start and noted the time on my alarm clock. It was 2 a.m. The breeze stopped just as fast as it had started. I got out of bed and put the screen back in place.

An hour later I got the phone call from my brother to say that my mother had died at 2 am. That screen had never blown out before, nor has it blown out since.

Charlene

Another woman was comforted by a message from the elements. Her mother, Edith, had lived with her for 30 years after Charlene's father died. For the last few years of her life, Edith needed round-the-clock care, which only a nursing home could provide. Charlene missed the final few days of her mother's life because of a vacation and was most upset that she hadn't been there when her mother actually died. Later she was taking her mother's ashes into the cemetery where her mother's parents and her husband lay buried. It was a gloomy, cloudy day.

The daughter came to her father's grave and found she could push back part of the gravestone and put her mother's ashes within. The minute she had done this, the sun came out and a beautiful rainbow was visible.

Charlene felt that her mother was very pleased and that, finally, for Charlene, was a sense of completion, the necessary conclusion.

Connections after the death

Crows and hummingbirds are the birds most often named as messengers. As soon as Susan died, several of us in her women's support group had visits from crows. Her closest friend saw two crows, which stayed, close to the house all the next day. They kept squawking at her. Not only that, but also three other people talked of crows around them the day after she died. I had noticed crows talking to me for days subsequent to her death, although at the time I hadn't made the connection with their appearance to Susan's death. Neither did I do so until the others mentioned crows.

The funeral

Some people claim a distinct impression of the sentiments of their loved one at the funeral.

Shirley

Shirley's husband died suddenly of a heart attack. She had seen his body just after his death in hospital and felt that it wasn't him at all. Without the spirit of the man who had shared her life for 20 years, the body was just an empty shell. In spite of contrary advice from her mother-in-law, she dressed him in a white shroud for his funeral and followed the formal steps required by their religion which had been seldom practiced. She explained that her husband Tim had been a deeply spiritual person although he had not focused much of his time on religion. So she followed her instincts and made the funeral arrangements accordingly. On the day of the funeral she thought his body looked wonderful and said he looked happy and ten years younger.

Sara

Sara stopped by the open casket of her best friend before the funeral began. While she stood quietly looking at the body, she felt the deceased make a request, urging her to, "Fix my hair!" She felt her friend was upset at what the undertaker had done to arrange her hair. So she found someone who would arrange the friend's hair she described to the dresser how the deceased would have done it herself.

When this was done it seemed as if the spirit of her friend was at peace and no longer concerned about her looks. Sara had never been open to any suggestion of such communication and was totally surprised at how strongly she felt the command.

I went to the funeral of a friend, which was a glorious ceremony; it included friends speaking from their hearts, playing instruments and singing specially written songs for her.

After the ceremony I went up to look into in the open casket. I looked at the body that was clearly devoid of life, and sensed a presence up in the left-hand corner of the room. I sensed her up there, seemingly much amused. I found myself smiling up into the corner of the room. She was just fine.

Special sign at the funeral

Frank

Frank died on hospice care. His wife Mary was a wonderful caretaker, though they were both sad to be parting after a long and wonderfully close marriage. Mary had asked him to send her a sign, if possible to say he was OK after his death if he possibly could. Mary told me the following.

His special gift to her had always been red roses. At his funeral, Mary noticed a very odd flower arrangement. Three dramatic red roses had been placed in a bouquet of quiet blue and white flowers. This she understood to be his sign to her, Mary felt the red roses represented their love and the quantity, three, each one of their children.

To the skeptic: we are not talking about the immaculate creation of red roses, but perhaps the florist had a sudden urge to place those roses there, or made a mistake. However, don't you wonder where those sudden impulses come from?

Sign from animals after the funeral

Cindy
After her father died Cindy watched her aging mother struggle to cope with life alone. When her mother became sick, Cindy cared for her with help from hospice. After a long and wretched illness Cindy's mother died. Despite her personal loss and natural grief Cindy was glad her mother was no longer suffering. After the funeral, she and her husband drove along a country road in the dark: they had to break sharply to avoid hitting two deer, which had decided to cross the road. Cindy saw the deer leap out, gamboling and frolicking, enjoying their freedom. One was a magnificent stag and the other smaller deer, a smaller doe. The stag was in the lead, but the doe stopped, highlighted in the car headlights and looked straight at Cindy who had an overwhelming feeling it was her mother, happy and gamboling with her father again.

That incident had a big impact on Cindy. She felt she had just received a clear message from her mother who was indicating to her that she was fine and was finally together again with her father. Inevitably, Cindy felt much more peaceful about her mother's death.

Special connections

Many people have reported a belief that they have had some contact with the deceased after their death. I have known people who have talked to the dying person who has agreed to send a sign after death if they possibly can. Often something that seems commonplace happens, but for the bereaved the event takes on special significance. Some people get this message themselves and others have used mediums. After hearing some details the deceased would have known, they are convinced that their loved one was contacted. Other people may have very vivid dreams, hear words, sounds or even sense smells and be convinced their loved one is trying to communicate with them. These reactions happen quite frequently. Sometimes the connection is just a quiet sense of, on the part of the recipient, peace or love. These connections may happen at any time in the first week or so, in the following weeks or months, or even years later.

In the support group I lead, I find people are reluctant to relate episodes about the signs they have been given from their deceased friends and relatives. They fear people will think they are insane, or at best a little crazy! I understand the reasons for their hesitancy completely; nevertheless, I can easily reassure them and encourage them to share their experience with the rest of the group if they so choose.

As soon as I say something to the effect, "That's quite a common type of experience and I truly believe you had that experience," others in the group start acknowledging similar experiences. I would guess at least fifty percent of the people I talk to have had some kind of experience of the above nature.

The strange thing is that desperately wanting to get some sign does not make it happen, and I have to be careful not to let people feel bad who don't get these kinds of experiences. Nearly everybody will agree there are times they experience a sudden, inexplicable sense of peace.

Ghosts?

Various sources, from the movie *Ghost* to Tibetan writings, talk of the soul taking time to move fully out of this world and into the next, so perhaps the energy of the departed is more available over a certain number of days after the death.

When I was eight years old, my Uncle Ben died. I remember being told how much my Uncle Ben loved me and he was said to be overjoyed when I was born. I remember his calling me his princess. He lived several hundred miles from us so I only saw him when we visited in the summer and at Christmas. I loved to visit my aunt, but I was scared of Uncle Ben. He was an alcoholic.

One summer day we received a telegram to say he had died. Darkness falls late in summer in England, so there was still light in my bedroom when later that evening I was lying in bed, but still wide awake. Plainly I saw a white translucent shape at the foot of my bed. I knew it was my Uncle. It was his size and shape although no details were apparent. I felt an absolute sense of comfort and love. I shall feel forever that he came to make peace and to leave me with no doubt of his true love for me.

I was old enough to know not to tell anyone this story, so no one would laugh at me. However, the experience certainly changed how I remembered my uncle Ben. Now I remember his love for me and forget my earlier fears.

One of my colleagues, for whom I felt respect died, without warning, of a heart attack. We had talked at length and both felt we were trying to make a positive difference in the world through our contribution in the workplace. He had offered great encouragement and support to quite a number of people. The news of his death spread rapidly at work, and many people were quite shocked because there had been no inkling of illness.

The day after his death, he came to me in a vision. His face was crystal clear and large, it filled my whole field of vision. He laughed at me and said "You have to carry the ball by yourself now."

The laugh left me with a feeling of friendly support. I was able to think, "Yes, maybe I am at a point where I no longer need his support and encouragement, and I can continue to help others." I felt empowered by the exchange.

Sense of presence

Many people tell me that they sense that their loved one is still where they were habitually. Other hospice bereavement coordinators tell me they have heard these kinds of stories more often than they can count.

Joe

Joe and his mother spent the evenings together watching TV. After his mother died, Joe said he would talk out loud to her about what was happening on TV, because he felt she was there sitting in her usual chair.

Helga

Helga's husband had died after a long fight with cancer. Shortly after the funeral she got rid of the living room furniture and bought a new set. She loved using the big armchair, but some evenings she didn't go and sit in it because she felt her husband was sitting there.

Gwendolyn

Katherine died when she was in her fifties. She had been on hospice and had been cared for by her daughter, Gwendolyn, in her home until she died. Gwen had been close to her mother. She had come to closure and felt complete, but of course she missed her mother. She did report that she often sensed her mother's presence and said her mother often made her presence known. I asked for some examples.

One day Gwen was sitting in her infant son's bedroom when she felt that the spirit of her mother was in the room. In her mind she said, "Well if you are here, then make your presence known." Immediately the child's mobile started moving, although no one was near to wind it up.

The second story Gwen told was of a visit to the zoo with her children. They were standing watching the polar bear enclosure, but they were next to the bear's pool and could see underwater through the window. The bears had a baby bear that was the cause of much interest. Hundreds of people encircled that enclosure. Gwen said in her mind, "Mom if you are there, please have the baby polar bear come up to my child." Within a couple of minutes that baby polar bear came right up to her child, stayed looking at him right in the eyes and blew bubbles at him in the water.

Gwen was thrilled by these events and continues to feel the comforting presence of her mother.

Jennifer

A woman, Marjorie, adopted an eleven-year-old girl Jennifer, late in her life. They had been extremely close for twenty years when the old lady died.

Jennifer said, " I feel my mother with me constantly."

This feeling of on-going connection is so helpful to many people in the earlier months of their loss. They feel loved and cared for, and they are convinced the spirit of their loved one lives on.

Gertrude

I was visiting a widow in her seventies, once a month for a few months. Her husband had died after an exhausting period of illness and home care. One day I went in her house and sat down to talk. She said she had nearly called me at home at 3 a.m. one morning. Of course I asked why and she said there had been a man in the house. So I asked if she had called the police, but she hadn't and had been glad later when she found all the doors and windows locked the next morning. She had been quite scared of this encounter. I asked questions and pieced together the story.

Gertrude had woken up from sleep because she heard a man's footsteps in her hall. She was about to get up to check the situation, but then he walked into her bedroom and said nothing. He walked to the end of the bed and stood looking at her. She couldn't see his features but he had curly hair and looked like her husband had looked when they first met.

Feeling the Feelings

Of course the process is different for everyone, and is influenced largely by the degree in which our lives were bound up with that of the deceased. A widow left alone after 50 years of a close marriage relationship will find it very hard to adjust to the bereavement. It can be so hard to even come to accept that the person is dead. In general, sudden death, which allows no time for any preparation whatever, either practical or emotional, is harder to come to terms with than one preceded by a prolonged illness. In later cases people are already grieving as the person is dying. In general it is harder to lose a spouse than a parent or sibling, and losing a child, no matter what their age is terrible. The frequency of interaction with the deceased is another big factor as is the length of the relationship.

The intense feelings of the bereaved can be totally overwhelming and yet the road to healing seems to require those feelings to be felt. Suppressing feelings in an attempt to be in control, may lead to physical and emotional problems later. So the task for the bereaved at this stage is to combine letting themselves feel the feelings without getting overwhelmed by them. Taking care of themselves becomes an equal priority. They will need to tack between feeling their feelings and taking care of themselves. In order to achieve a balance between looking after their physical and mental well being and necessary healthy grieving, it may mean setting time aside to do one, then the other. Self-caring also includes asking for help. It may be a struggle to even get out of bed in the morning. Devastated survivors may not be convinced that life is worth living.

Grieving people need someone who will be there just to listen. The last thing they need is someone telling them why they should cheer up, why they should be grateful, why they should count their blessings, or worst of all hear that it was God's will. Theories are fine, but each person walks this path alone and in his own way. The best we can do is listen and care, which helps a great deal. The bereaved with family and friends that stand by on good days and on bad days are fortunate. That support is crucial.

Support groups and grief counselors are available to those who need it. The cost of visiting counselors may be covered by insurance, and hospices across the country offer free bereavement support groups, open to the public.

As a hospice bereavement coordinator I make a call to the bereaved about a week after the death and visit if they want me to or if the nurses think it would be desirable. So I listen to many stories. Often they cry and sometimes I weep a few tears, too. So far I think in every first visit of an hour or so, that I have made, we have laughed at some point as well as cried.

Dreams

Grace

An elderly hospice patient told me about her husband's death 25 years earlier. She had been totally devastated. They had been very close for over 40 years. She had relied on him for support in many ways. When her husband died Grace had to face the loss of her home, learn to drive, write a check and cope with all the other complexities of day-to-day life alone. Until his death her husband had done all those things for her.

Grace told me of a very vivid dream she had a few months after her husband's death. In this dream her husband came to her and said, "It's time to stop your crying and get on with your life. You will never know how much I love you, but when it's your time to leave, I am going to reach down and lift you up to be with me."

Grace said she had shared her dream with people at the time it occurred and they were very skeptical about it and said it was just in her imagination. I assured her that I believed that the dream would come true. That was such a comfort to her as she approached her own death.

Matthew

A friend counseled an elderly man called Matthew, who had lost his wife after 56 years of marriage. He felt the loss terribly and said that he felt he could come to some measure of peace if he just knew she was all right. As he was lying down in bed at night he would repeat to himself his willingness to receive a message. He described a dream.

"My wife was standing across the room facing my bed. She was looking at me and smiling. She walked toward the left side of my bed and stroked my arm very lovingly. I can still feel her touch."

That was the sign the man had hoped for. He felt his prayer had been answered; he knew she was all right, that their love lived on. He came to some degree of peace and was able to set aside his pain and hold on to their love and his happy memories.

Helen

Helen's husband of 58 years died of cancer. She felt she was coping pretty well with her bereavement, though she missed him terribly because they had done everything together. A few weeks after he died she had a beautiful dream that she described to me.

"We were walking together along this country road in the fall. We always loved to walk together and we had walked in similar places around here and in Maine. The trees were beautiful and the leaves were falling. Then I noticed one tree that hadn't lost its leaves. I kept trying to get his attention and point out the tree with all its leaves."

The dream had been a wonderful connection for her, it brought back to her memory all the happy times they had spent walking together. Then she talked about the tree with all its leaves and drew the conclusion that they had both expected her to die over 10 years ago and to leave him. The fact that she was still alive was the mystery and wonder.

Charlene

Charlene's husband had died of a sudden heart attack and a few weeks after his death she had this dream.

She was at an event in a large auditorium with a number of her friends. She suddenly saw her husband sitting in a different area. This seemed perfectly normal and natural to her and she called over to him, "Honey don't you want to come over and sit with us?" and he replied, "No I'm okay over here."

The message Charlene took from the dream was that he was fine but now his place was "over there."

Jane

Jane's husband of thirty years had been dead for several

months before she dreamt the following:

"I dreamed of us being together again in our favorite vacation spot, we were in the very room we had stayed in many times. He told me that although he could visit me, I shouldn't tell my mother or anyone else."

It appeared that his connection to Jane was such that he could visit her in her dreams, but not reach other people.

Norman

Norman's wife of forty years had been dead for a few months when he had this dream.

She was telling him she wanted to come back, but Norman had been through so much pain in trying to accept her death he said, "No you can't come back now. I couldn't deal with the pain of losing you all over again."

As he thought about the dream later, Norman was comforted because he felt that his wife still cared deeply about him and wanted to be with him still.

Patricia

Patricia dreamt of her dead husband Paul.

I called my home and he answered the phone. I asked whether he would still be there when I got home and he said, "Maybe."

Sarah

On his birthday, Sarah dreamt of her deceased husband.

The setting was at night. She was returning home after visiting friends and saw something silver glittering in the gutter, she went over and picked it up. It was a beautiful Gucci watch.

Sarah felt this dream gave her a beautiful gift and spoke to her of the time of his birthday.

Lunar moth

Lunar moths are rare, extraordinarily large and quite beautiful. Many people have never even seen one. One or more lunar moths came to visit three people after a member, a graceful, well-loved lady died after a lengthy illness.

A few weeks after the funeral, her husband visited her grave and noticed a lunar moth on her gravestone. A week later her sister-in-law visited her grave and a lunar moth hovered around her. A few days after that, her 6 year-old grandson called his mother to see the lunar moth that was dancing around him, and he told his mother that he knew the moth was his grandmother.

One sighting of a lunar moth is interesting and unusual. Three sightings within the same family, seem to be more than a coincidence and the family believed that this was a communication from their loved one.

Roses

Sheila

Sheila was totally devastated by her husband's death. They had had a long and close relationship. After his death, her family was very concerned about her, but she couldn't bring herself to spend much time with people, she preferred to be alone with her memories.

One day Sheila's house was suddenly filled with a scent of roses, a scent that both she and her husband had loved. It occurred a second time when her brother was present. It was unmistakable and no rational cause could be found.

Sheila was convinced that the smell was a sign from her husband, both a message that he was all right and that he watched and cared about her still. He used to buy roses for her often. Sheila was comforted by the connection considerably.

Kathleen

Kathleen had a very good relationship with her mother. She had been able to support her dying mother at home with hospice help, and was content that she had done everything she could for her until death. Of course she missed her mother dearly as they had been very close. An old friend of the family gave Kathleen a picture of a deep pink rose, with dark green leaves, inscribed with the words: *I will be with you always*. The gift was special because of the sentiment and the thoughtfulness of the friend, but the experiences that followed were quite a surprise.

Kathleen said she was an avid gardener and had planted every single thing in her garden over twenty years, so nothing escaped her attention. She looked out of her kitchen door and saw a deep pink rose growing by a stonewall. She knew no rose had been growing there before. She walked over to it and saw the rose was the same deep pink of the painting. A few days later Kathleen checked out some new roses she had planted the previous year. One was meant to be a white rose, tipped with green and the other a vivid red. When each of these roses bloomed they were replicas of those on the plate.

The blooms on all three rose bushes matched the deep pink in the painting. Kathleen felt that she was receiving a clear message from her mother telling her that she was indeed still with her.

Kevin

Kevin's father had been a keen gardener and a rose lover. The old man had planted a row of six climbing roses before he got sick. Like the old man the roses grew wanly and died. Kevin didn't bother to dig out the roots, but planted new roses in front of the dead ones. Three years later, the old man got sicker and finally died one day in February.

Later that year, in early summer, Kevin noticed that all the dead roses planted by his father came back to life and flowered.

Kevin took that sign of roses coming to life as a communication from his father. He felt it was a message telling him of a continuation of his father's life, in a different form.

Other signs

Rachel

Rachel's husband had been dead for two months, when she had this experience.

One morning she got out of bed and noticed an indentation in the bed next to her spot, as if someone had been sleeping there next to her. She understood that to be a sign from her husband. Rachel was another person to be greatly comforted by this sign of caring and connection from her husband.

John

John was totally distraught by his wife's death. He wanted to be alone and planned on going away for a few days. His family was worried for his safety, so his sister was trying to persuade him not to go away. She was anxious about him concerned about him and felt he would be safer around people.

John argued determinedly with his sister that he needed time alone, away from people as part of his healing process. Suddenly his sister became very hot, uncomfortably so. As a result she stopped arguing with her brother, felt normal again and was prepared to help him.

John felt he knew what was best for him and needed his sister's sanction and support in pursuing an action he felt was best for him. The sister was of course amazed that such a thing could happen. John and his wife had believed strongly in a life after death and he felt very comforted. It seemed that his wife continued to be looking out for him in some form or other, and it seemed to him to offer proof that their love continued.

Visits in dreams
Death of children is hard to accept no matter what the age. We all assume that the oldest die first, so we think that we will die before our children. Most of those children, who die so young, seem to have been very special. I have heard people describe them as angels who came for a short visit.

Marcia
Marcia had a beautiful daughter who had cancer at an early age and, after a prolonged illness, died at the age of ten. Someone else who had known her described her as, "one of those angels." She had some mystery about her, and was pretty, thoughtful, and good in school. She was every parent's dream of a child. Naturally, her mother was totally devastated by her daughter's death.

On several different occasions Marcia had dreams that included a visit from her daughter. Sin her dreams Marcia was so thrilled to see her young daughter again, but every time she went to hug her, her daughter disappeared and Marcia woke up with a start, realizing it was just a dream and she would never be able to give her daughter that hug again in the flesh.

Marcia just loved the dreams, although she felt intensely the anguish of not being able to hug her daughter. Nevertheless the dreams seemed real always, moreover, she felt sure the dream were messages to tell her that her daughter was fine. Marcia found these messages very comforting.

Andrea

Andrea had four children, the eldest one died at the age of 19 in a car driven off the road by a peer at summer school. The event was traumatic not only because her daughter had died, but also because of the way it had happened which was very hard to accept. The two families even knew each other and the driver of the car survived the crash.

Subsequently, Andrea had a dream where she saw her daughter just standing there looking straight at her. Then she smiled at her mother and said that she was okay, and then turned away, stepped up and took a bear's outstretched helping paw in her hand. Later Andrea discovered that in Native American lore the bear's paw is taken to be the hand of God.

A few weeks later at a memorial service for her daughter, the mother of the girl who had driven the car came up to Andrea with a small gift. She said, "I don't know why, but I just felt compelled to buy you this." Andrea opened the present and found a small leather pouch with an Indian motif on it. She pulled open the drawstring pouch and pulled out a very small piece of jade. The carving on the jade was of a bear!

Then Andrea told the donor of the gift, the dream and explained the significance of the bear. It was such a clear message to Andrea that her daughter was at peace and with God, that it gave her an enormous sense of peace. She carries that pouch in her pocketbook everywhere she goes.

Mechanical equipment

Mary Lee's husband had died and subsequently Mary Lee visited a psychic to talk about her life in general and her next steps. The psychic had a practice of leaving a tape recorder running as she spoke. She conveyed to Mary Lee that her husband wanted to be able to communicate with her. Mary Lee responded that she was open to that and would try to listen.

The psychic talked with Mary Lee at length and left the tape recorder running the whole time. Later Mary Lee replayed the tape. When she heard herself say to the psychic that she would be open to hearing from her dead husband, she heard, "Mean it," in a man's voice superimposed on the tape.

She was convinced this was her husband trying to communicate with her. Later she was able to do some automatic writing that she was convinced came via her husband. This communication from her dead husband was a tremendous comfort to her.

Summary

Numerous stories tell of occurrences beyond what we normally accept as real. They seem to occur at the moment people most need to hear them. Events such as these convince people that there is something beyond our everyday experience, beyond our physical world, and that their loved one is all right and at peace. Such experiences provide an enormous measure of comfort to a great number of people.

Often we are too busy to listen, and when we are in pain we keep even busier to distract ourselves from pain. That's why so many events happen when people are half asleep or just in a dream. When people are asleep, the mind has shut down enough to allow other things to get through. If people desire to get some kind of communication they have to be still. They must take time to be quiet in thought as well as action. They might suggest they are open to a special dream just before they go to sleep at night.

Knowing that this is possible, that these connections are common is a relief to most people. The fact they have control over whether they wish them to continue or stop is an even greater relief to them. I have told people of all ages who are troubled by such experiences that they can talk to the image or vision of the person, and explain they are fine, and that it's time for the spirit to leave them now, and go on to what they need to do next. This has worked in all cases I've dealt with so far.

Once the bereaved achieve some degree of acceptance of their loss they will no longer search for signs or messages. They no longer need the person who died to be spending time around them.

The Grieving Process

Uniqueness

Everyone is unique and is going to grieve in his own way and in his own time. There are models of grief, which can be very helpful to survivors. It is quite a relief and a comfort to find your symptoms and experiences are relatively normal. Sometimes a bereaved person needs to get more help, as his losses are overwhelming, which is frequently true for people have who have experienced multiple losses, or who have extenuating circumstances.

During my training in grief counseling, I listened to a woman talk about her very painful experience. The tension in the room was palpable, and one person asked a question about tools and techniques, most probably to relieve their own tension. The vehement response from the woman in pain was, "I just needed a real human being who would listen!" I knew then, I could do this job. Family and friends also can be what the bereaved person needs, if they are willing to listen, to be truly present, and to share her pain for a while.

When the impending death is acknowledged ahead of time,

then loved ones may grieve ahead of the death. I spoke to one woman who said that she is no longer afraid of death, that the process of being there with her father as he was dying was truly beautiful. Loved ones who have had the opportunity to stand witness in this way, are truly enriched. They will grieve their loss, but their lives have already been transformed, and they will move forward with the love and the happy memories from that relationship.

Typical passages

Dr Ross's model of loss describes the process of grief quite well. Initially someone may be in shock, and denial, unable to believe his loved one is really dead and won't be returning. This is a way of protecting himself from a reality he isn't ready to face. A woman may organize a reception after her husband's funeral and company may say, "Look how well she is doing, she's not breaking down." She may not be doing well at all; she may just be numb, functioning on automatic pilot, and going through the customary motions of living. The task, in this phase of grief, is to accept the death and to know that the person will not come back.

In the second phase, the bereaved does understand only too well that her loved one will not return, and she can feel all sorts of emotions intensely. She may feel sadness, loneliness, guilt, anger and a host of other emotions. Her task now is to both let herself feel her feelings, and to take care of herself. This will mean asking for help, too.

Then depression can hit very hard. People describe how they feel. They say, they can't understand how the world goes on normally, when the bottom has just fallen out of their world. They may not even be able to get out of bed in the morning and get dressed.

Eventually the survivors come full circle to acceptance of the death, and slowly begin to have renewed energy to reinvest in life again. No one knows how much time it will take. I have seen a woman in denial for a year, I have seen a woman feeling intense emotions 4 years later, and I have seen a woman, who suffered her loss intensely, reinvesting in life after months not years.

This model is not so linear as it sounds. The bereaved can go through all stages in a cycle, from shock to acceptance in a day, and repeat the whole cycle the next day. They can feel they move forward for 3 days, then slide back and feel terrible again.

I always encourage bereaved persons to see their doctor. They may need medication for a short period to help them get enough sleep, and if they get terribly depressed, they may also need medication to give them a base level they won't fall below. Survivors having symptoms of ailments, may have put their own needs on hold for a long time while caring for their loved one, or may be experiencing symptoms that have more to do with their emotional state.

Processing grief can look very different. One person may cry and cry, another may be quiet and solitary, while another may continue as normal wondering why everything seems to go wrong around them.

I do believe that unresolved grief causing an enormous number of problems and issues. I know a woman who was in a car crash shortly after her husband died. I know a man who got violent and attacked a doctor for "letting" his wife die. I know a woman who lost her job shortly after her mother died. I know a woman who developed severe asthma after her husband died. The list goes on.

Occasionally I meet a person who can change when I point out the connection between loss and their physical state. I was talking on the phone one day with a woman and I could hear the difficulty she was having breathing. She told me her lung problems started right after her husband's death. I said, "Do you know the Taoists believe that we hold grief in our lungs?" She was silent for a moment, but when she started talking, she was breathing much more easily. I'm not sure which one of us was the more surprised!

So grief takes many forms, depending on the bereaved person himself and on the nature of the relationship that he had with the deceased.

Bereavement support from hospice

One of the services that hospice provides is on-going support to the family who survives the person who was care for by hospice. That is true whether the person died at home, in a hospice residence or in a nursing home. The coverage lasts through the first year's anniversary. The exact nature of support will vary with the individual hospice, but in general will include: one or more visits, phone calls, mailings, support groups, and a memorial service. Accreditation for hospice includes a requirement that hospices maintain contact with the survivors and make help available. The balance of professional and volunteer help may vary, and hospices develop programs to meet the needs of their local communities.

The bereavement coordinator participates in the hospice team meetings, so is well aware of the history of the patient under hospice care, and of the family situation. The social worker, spiritual coordinator and nurse have shared the step-by-step adjustments the family was making, and the team discussed their concerns about the family's ability to cope after the death occurs. Collectively the team decides how best to support them. The families themselves, though, make the decision about what support they will accept.

Within a few days of the death, the nurse will visit or call the survivor. Sometimes the social worker goes back to visit, too. As a bereavement coordinator, I call her between 7 and 10 days later. I aim to call when the visitors who came for the funeral have just left, and the bereaved is alone for the first time. The survivors have probably been extremely busy and overwhelmed with company, and have had little time to let the reality sink in. I offer to visit each family, but if the team thinks the family really needs help, I say I am coming, what time would suit you? More people decline than accept a visit, but quite a few let me call back a month later. I like to do this, because the bereaved person may still be numb after a week and think she is coping, but time can bring significant changes. So I go from month to month. When the person is feeling all right, she won't want to spend time talking to me, and that is fine. Quite a few people would like me calling monthly for life, but I try to get each one to use other resources, so she is comfortable when I need to stop the hospice support 12 months after her loss.

Visits

When I go to visit, I am there to listen and to give guidance. I may shed a few tears with the griever if she cries, but every time I've visited, we have laughed together, too. I can confirm her process and support her decisions, let her know what's normal and typical, and make suggestions of what might be helpful at this stage of her grief.

I do suggest going to a therapist, even weekly for a while, to anyone really struggling to deal with her loss, and who does not have really good support from family and friends.

If the family had a regular volunteer visiting to relieve the caretaker when the person was dying, I ask that volunteer to go visit the family again a few times. Volunteers frequently have become close to the family, helping at such a tough time in their life, so the family welcomes them back. I remember being very surprised at a party the family gave after the death of a mother, who they had supported for a long time. I seemed to be almost a guest of honor. I had spent time there as a volunteer, quietly sitting with the old lady each Saturday afternoon, and I hadn't realized how much I was appreciated.

Suggestions pop into my head without any logical reason. I give the survivor the suggestion, surprising us both, as it is spot on. I've suggested creating a memorial garden, or a specific short cut way of journaling ideas that were immediately accepted.

I really enjoy these visits. I know I can make a difference by accepting her sadness and loneliness, yet bringing in new hope of better times.

Calls

At my initial call at 7 to 10 days after the death, I offer to call again in 4 weeks. Most people will accept this offer, because neither of us knows how they will be feeling by them. I continue calling monthly if the survivor wants me to. So many of those calls are personally rewarding. A woman's low monotone voice may just answer "Hello," but when I tell them who it is, her voice will lift, "Oh Margaret! How are you?" There is nothing like making someone's day! This enables me to keep in touch with far more people than I would ever have time to visit, and also to stay in touch with family members who are in different parts of the country.

Many times follow-up calls are made by specially trained hospice volunteers. We use a volunteer to call at 6 months, even if the survivor had said he was coping fine earlier, and didn't feel need for close attention. They always seem to appreciate the volunteer's interest and phone call. Some hospices have volunteers make calls on key anniversaries like birthdays and wedding anniversaries.

Mailings

Hospices provide mailings to the bereaved families, which vary in the details, but follow much the same pattern as I follow. I send a bereavement card out within the first week, and a letter at 4 weeks with enclosures of a simple booklet, a list of therapists, a list of support groups and a bibliography. Four weeks seems to be about the right time. A bereaved person's attention span tends to be so limited in those early days, that he may ignore or mislay mail.

Hospice volunteers do a great job of getting out subsequent mailings. We send a letter with enclosures at 3 months and at 6 months after the death, and a handwritten card at 9 months and 13 months. We also send information just before the holidays, and in the final card, to suggest ways to cope with holidays, and that first year anniversary. Sometimes a survivor will mail back to the volunteer to say how much he appreciated the card.

Support groups

All hospices offer support groups to the bereaved family and friends of the deceased hospice patients. These support groups are available to the public at large, free of charge, as part of the hospice's community service. In urban communities there will be sufficient numbers of people to run specialized groups, such as: death of a parent both for adults and children, death of a spouse, or death of a child. A number of organizations exist to support specific types of loss e.g. Compassionate Friends for loss of a child.

Usually these hospice provided groups, will be advertised in local newspapers and the hospice families will be notified by mail. Anyone looking for a group can call a local hospice number they find in the phone book.

The leader needs some training and experience, to run a group well. I do find if I can be present and in my heart, then the group seems to manage itself. Support groups are not right for everyone. When each person is willing to be there for each other, to listen and contribute when it feels appropriate, then the group gains so much from each other, the leader is hardly needed. Some people may find it helpful to be there and listen without talking much at all. Some grievers are better served by a personal therapist, when they have so many issues, that they need to talk a full hour.

Many times I have been amazed to see the nature of the losses of people coming to an open general group. Some times the group has been comprised totally of women, sometimes totally of men, and sometimes each member has suffered the same type of loss. Each person's situation and feelings provide insight for the others. The agenda seems to have been formulated elsewhere, unknown to us all, when we see the commonalities and contrasts in the people presenting themselves.

Memorial service

Hospices also provide an annual or bi-annual service of remembrance and celebration. Different hospices organize this in different ways, to meet the needs of their local community. Perhaps only 10 % of hospice families avail themselves of this program, but those who do attend are usually very appreciative.

Hospice personnel can also be called on to help in their community in times of loss. I have talked in schools, in senior centers, to church groups, and on cable TV in giving guidance on dealing with loss. Other hospices may do far more.

Special Experiences

I have already shared some of the special experiences that bereaved people have described to me, close to the time of the actual death. These experiences can relieve some of their grief. Now they can believe in a connection to something beyond this life, and they can interpret the experience, as a sign that their loved one is fine, and they live on is some form we don't understand. Those sorts of experiences seem to come to the people who are ready to face their loss and are open to receiving a message in that way.

Many times the bereaved will tell me that they feel the presence of their loved ones with them most of the time. Grief is not about letting go; it's about finding ways to integrate your history, to take the ongoing love, and to take the happy memories with you into your future.

Reinvesting in Life

What we have once enjoyed and deeply loved we cannot lose; for all that we love deeply becomes a part of us. —Helen Keller [*11]

In loss, bereaved people cannot imagine their pain will one day lessen. Nevertheless, time does heal, though no one can tell how much time each individual requires for the healing process. I've heard people say they were going through the motions of life without any real enjoyment, they "fake it 'til they make it." Then one day they noticed they did something they actually enjoyed and didn't think of their loss for a while. Gradually, once they felt comfortable talking to people again they found they could return to doing more of the things they used to enjoy. Slowly they began to make a new life for themselves. That doesn't mean that they wouldn't love to go back to the life they once had, but slowly they begin to adjust to a different situation and construct a new life for themselves.

The following stories are from people who are getting on with their lives in one way or another. Death of their loved one is no longer a primary issue in their minds but some experience reminds them of their connection to the departed. Some of the experiences were comforting and some were truly life changing. They do suggest the on-going connection stays for a lifetime.

Visits of the spirit

My father died when I was 40. The event triggered my own mid life crisis as I began to sort out who I was when I was without that relationship. After my father's death, I went through therapy and saw the relationship with my father more clearly, both the good and the bad. I had worked through my early feelings of anger at his absence when I was small.

Four or five years later I was in a meditation group and saw a very clear vision of my father saying he wanted to talk to me. (My visions are crystal clear, although I don't see that clearly normally.) I wasn't about to take in that energy myself, having worked so hard not to let his beliefs and assumptions drive my behavior. After the session I told the leader about my vision, and she said, "Oh he's here now. He says to tell you that you are going to be all right, that your mother is okay, and that you will see her in three weeks time." (The leader had no way of knowing that I would be seeing my mother in exactly three weeks.) She added, "He just came to tell you he loves you." As she spoke I could feel my father's presence and a special energy penetrated my skin by about half an inch. I felt at peace. Everything became crystal clear to me and I am happy in the knowledge that it was a peaceful resolution and the appropriate closure of our relationship.

In this new and comfortable state of awareness, I drove home, suddenly I found I could sing. I must emphasize that all my family tells me that singing is very definitely not one of my strengths. I walked into the living room, told my husband I could sing and promptly did so. He said on a scale of 1 to 10, I was normally a 2 but this singing was an 8. Neither of us could understand it and within 24 hours the ability faded.

It wasn't until several weeks later that I put two and two together and made the connection between my sudden gift of song and the visit of my father. I felt I was given something demonstrable to prove to me there was something there, which I could call real. Again this event brought me peace over both my father's death and on the impact he had on me as a developing child.

Chas

Once a month for a year I joined a group that was meditating on world peace. The leader was a joyous, jubilant man, generous in girth and spirit named Chas. He was very much in touch with the call of spirit, of love and empowerment. Successfully, he facilitated workshops for people to see the wondrous side of themselves.

Unfortunately the world wasn't quite ready to pay sufficiently for his services, so he struggled with some of the practical aspects of the physical world. He loved so many people, and so many people loved him. Furthermore, he also loved food and knew he could have been kinder to his physical body.

Chas was only in his forties when he had a sudden heart attack and died instantly. His funeral was particularly special with many attendees. Amongst these was an old friend who delivered a glowing tribute to him and an honest appraisal for a eulogy.

Several years later his widow, Allison, recounted this story of a visit from Chas.

"Last month I was lying in my bed in our apartment and Chas just appeared sitting on the edge of the bed. He was wearing a white robe. I felt quite calm and asked him what he had been doing since he left. He said something like he had been in school learning how to take care of himself. He said he was learning the things that I had tried to get him to do when he was here. He said something about my not needing to carry on his work."

Allison had been waiting for such a sign from Chas. Knowing the intensity of the spiritual connection he had felt when alive she felt sure he would eventually find a way to communicate with her. Thus she came to a newfound peace. Many friends, too, were fascinated to hear what Chas was up to in a life beyond.

Channeled writing

One woman from our woman's group, Diane, had been a very close friend of Susan's for years. When Susan died Diane felt that she was supposed to keep a connection with her and that this would somehow be made possible. A psychic had suggested Diane try automatic writing. Consequently, Diane bought a special journal and a purple pen similar to the one that Susan had always used. Diane sat quietly and emptied her mind and eventually found that she could start writing. She had no idea what she was writing at the time, but when she read it through afterward it seemed clear that this was a message coming from Susan. Among other things Susan "dictated" about how it was beautiful where she was, but she had a job to do which was to work with children.

When the remaining group met for a weekend, Diane wrote page after page of Susan's communication early on the Sunday morning.

Diane read her writing to the group. There were special words to each one of us, both celebratory comments and advice on our next steps. At one point Diane read Susan's words: "I am in the hummingbird, God is in the hummingbird." Within minutes a hummingbird came to the window and hovered longer than I have ever seen a hummingbird hover. He flew farther along the window and hovered again. He seemed to get a look at each one of us in turn and bow his head.

That was the first hummingbird seen by anyone of us that year, and it was the first time the homeowner had ever seen a hummingbird at that location. Each one of us felt we were in connection with the divine. We had no doubts about that. Still, I wear the hummingbird pin we bought as a reminder of the occasion!

Other cultures

On the whole our American culture teaches us to rely on a scientific approach to life. We are rational, logical, believe in the miracles of modern technology therefore issues of death and spirit are very far from our acceptance and understanding. This is not necessarily so in other cultures. In some parts of the world death can be viewed quite differently. The specific religion practiced in any culture provides the framework with which they live. Not only do they accept death as part of life much better than we do in this country, they are open to concepts of spirits and on-going connections.

Many people celebrate a "Day of the Dead." The whole family takes a picnic to the cemetery and people dress up the tombs and generally have a good time whilst remembering their ancestors. Why not? What a great way to be remembered.

I had an opportunity to visit a Peruvian Quichuan family living in an old Inca stone house. In the one and only room there was an arched niche in the wall, and there, in the position of honor was a skull with a lit candle adjacent. We asked our guide and interpreter questions about it. The skull was that of the wife's mother. After the body had been buried for 3 years, their custom was to dig it up and bring it into the house. There it was revered. The adults would confer with it and ask advice and guidance from it, and felt they received it. The skull was used to baby sit when necessary. The grandchildren still believed that grandma was watching and they had better be good.

What a wonderful way to feel continuity within the family. Both adults and children believed their relative took a new form, but believed that she continued to be just as concerned about the surviving family's welfare after her death as she was in life.

At eighteen, my daughter spent a summer as a counselor at a summer camp. She and another girl her age lived with and supported twelve eight-year-old girls in a cabin. One child, a beautiful Puerto Rican, was having a hard time sleeping in this hut in the woods.

My daughter talked to her to try and understand how best to help her. The girl was happy to explain that at home the spirit of her dead grandmother would sit in her rocking chair bedside her bed every night and her presence gave the girl a warm sense of feeling of security. At camp there was no rocking chair and no spirit of her grandmother and she missed her! This was perfectly normal to that child and her family, and the sense she had of her grandmother's love and the constant connection and security that provided for her didn't disappear with her grandmother's death.

The treatment of the remaining body can be very different in some cultures. The Indian method was to set alight a funeral pyre and scatter the ashes in the holy Ganges River. Tibetans performed sky burials, where the body was ceremonially divided and fed to vultures. Both these cultures clearly saw the body as the unneeded shell that remains after the spirit has departed.

Suicide

Many religions used to considered suicide to be a serious offense. These days, suicide tends to be viewed in a more compassionate light; it is seen as an act taken as a result of deep stress or mental imbalance. Religions such as Roman Catholicism and Judaism have relaxed their refusal to give suicide victims a normal burial. Hinduism and Buddhism teach that the person who has committed suicide will have an unfortunate rebirth.

In the circumstance of suicide, the grief of the survivors is severe. Often they often tremendous guilt and wonder what they might have been able to do to prevent their loved one taking their own life. The examples of suicide in my own experience are as follows. One young man I knew at college committed suicide; I had even said no to his request for a date a couple of months before his death. At the time it was natural for me to wonder if, by accepting that date, I could have made a difference to him and helped him want to live. A man at work died suddenly, without us ever being told how he died, and we were left to suspect an act of suicide. As his manager, I had to wonder if I could have provided more support. In my role as a bereavement coordinator, I have tried to support three different people, each of whom had a child take their own life.

In hospice we see dying as a final stage of growth, therefore I don't see any room for the justification of suicide. My sense of the people I knew or heard about directly who committed suicide, was one of a deep anguish and emotional pain in their circumstances, which they were unable to face. I can only feel compassion and trust that their "God" is deeply loving. The bereaved, left in their wake, need all our understanding and compassion, too.

Summary
All these stories continue to demonstrate the on-going connection between the living and the dead. In particular they are interesting because the receivers of these experiences were already moving on with their lives. For them the pain of loss had receded and they were no longer looking for signs or connections. The experiences seemed to have happened to give the bereaved a sense of completion.

To reiterate, our American culture is so focused on the scientific, on the practical and on the physical, we routinely dismiss these kinds of stories. Some other cultures accept the concept of spirit or energy continuing after death, and that the love and concern for loved ones lives on. We are so often told it's just in our minds or in our imagination. Maybe it is. But maybe we need a new definition of "mind" and of "imagination."

Summary

We all experience losses in this life. Is it the lows in life that make the high so blissful? Maybe we know joy because we have known pain. Facing our pain, rather than running from it, seems to enable our hearts to break open rather than break down. Does it take heartbreak to make us open our hearts and develop compassion? Compassion is when we touch another's pain with our love. Pity is when we touch another's pain with our fear.

For much of our time we are busy. Busy with the demands of this life, and then busy because we have forgotten how to be any other way. Busyness is a great distraction to hold us from looking at things we don't want to look at. Dying brings us all to the keen essence of life. We no longer have time for distractions. Nothing could be more real than a limit on the years, months, and even days of a lifetime or a relationship.

In such times of both physical and emotional pain, people talk of the intensity of the love and the living they crammed into the time which remained for them. People working with the dying often hear, "We did more living in those last six months than in the rest of our lives together."

The blessings of moving through a conscious dying process

can be enormous. Medical attention can be directed toward making them as comfortable and as pain free as possible. When the dying have worked through their ties to life, they can say they are sorry, too, and ask forgiveness of others. They can forgive others, whether the recipients of this forgiveness know or not. It is important for the dying to tell people of their love for them, and so say goodbye, then they can truly depart peacefully. There is an enormous gift left for survivors, too. As they grew themselves to cope with the reality of an approaching death, and came to closure on unfinished business, they could share their love. Even when there are mixed feelings in a relationship, like letting go of the hurt, and accepting what is, everyone's healing can be facilitated. There is a strong sense of coming to closure for everyone

I have no doubt and many people would agree with me, that being with people who are dying is walking on the edge of this world and the next. We see and experience things that we can't explain. For all concerned the incredible love that can be experienced by some people in those last stages, is way beyond what we feel in our normal course of life.

The survivors, too, in participating in this process, know that no matter how much they will miss the person, their dying was as good as it could have been. In general, the survivors, whose loved ones have died with hospice support, tend to have an easier time in the process of bereavement. Usually they had no option but to acknowledge that death was approaching and had to begin to accept what was coming. They did have the comfort of knowing that they provided the care that fulfilled the dying person's wishes to die at home, and did everything they could to make them as comfortable as possible in their chosen environment. They knew that the processes of dying, although painful emotionally and physically, were as good as it gets.

Grief is a process, too. If we try to hide from it, we place some limits on how we will function in life. It is a process that takes as long as it takes. The bereaved cycle through disbelief, feeling the painful loss, and slowly beginning to reinvest in life. They need support from friends and family, from people who can express their own compassion and be there when needed. It can be a slow process to recreate a life that no longer includes the loved one in a physical sense. That life may not be what the survivor would have chosen, however it may evolve into something loving and extremely rewarding.

The false advice of "Let go" or "Put it behind you," may leave the bereaved struggling to do the impossible. When ready they find ways to take the past with them into their future. The people they loved already have had a major influence on their life, and the essence of what they valued in them lives on through them. Children continue more than the family name, they take forward values and build on the dreams and aspirations of their parents.

We Americans can learn from the cultures that take forward a way of bringing their deceased loved ones into their future. Conversations and shared memories are wonderful. Even if the conversation is upsetting and we cry together, it is a blessing for the pain is shared and we make room for the good memories and laughter. Slowly the pain memories recede and people can recall more of the good memories

Once the pain has passed, it is most pleasant to be surrounded with reminders of people who they knew loved them. As I look around my house, I count many connections: the grandmother clock, the vases, the paintings, the pottery, the jewelry, a stone, all connections to family and friends who are no longer visible.

The stories I have shared bring many of these experiences to light. The feelings of wonder and amazement help so many accept what is happening, they can take comfort in the belief that the essence of their loved one lives on in some form. These stories cross boundaries of religions; they are experiences that can happen to believers in an afterlife and to non-believers.

Love is our connection, and love can extend beyond any time and place. Love is truly all there is. The experiences that have come to so many people have provided great comfort to them, and I hope just the possibility of them being true brings comfort to a good many more. Remember anything can happen.

Notes

*1 *New and Selected Poems*, by Mary Oliver, copyright© 1992 by Mary Oliver. Reprinted by permission by Beacon Press, Boston.

*2 From *LETTERS TO A YOUNG POET* by Ranier Maria Wilke, translated by Stephen Mitchell. Used by permission by Random House, Inc.

*3 Based on Elisabeth Kubler-Ross' model of the stages a dying person goes through before he can accept the fact that he is dying.

*4 Five Wishes Document, *Aging with Dignity*, Tallahasse, FL; Call 1-888-5WISHES (1-888-594-7437).

*5 Jerome Groopman, MD, Chief of Experimental Medicine, gave a talk, "Facing Mortality: Preserving One's Humanity and Hope," to the President's Circle at Beth Israel Deaconess Medical Center, June 16th 1998.

*6 Lachlan Farrow, MD, Director of the Palliative Care Program at Beth Israel Deaconess Medical Center, gave a talk to doctors and staff at Deaconess-Nashoba Medical Center, January 21st 2003.

*7 Extract From Emmanuel's Book II by Pat Rodegast & Judith Stanton, copyright© 1989 by Pat Rodegast and Judith

Stanton. Used by permission of Bantam Books, a division of Random House, Inc.

*8 Dame Cecily Saunders, "I Was Sick and You Visited Me," Christian Nurse International, 3, no. 4 (1987).

*9 Stephen Levine, interviewed by Peggy Roggenbuck, *New Age Magazine*, September 1979, 50.

*10 Sogyal Rinpoche, *The Tibetan Book of Living and Dying*. HarperSanFransico, New York 1989, 224.

*11 Quote from Helen Keller reprinted by courtesy of the American Foundation of the Blind, Helen Keller Archives.

Suggested Reading

Alborn, Mitch. *Tuesdays with Morrie*
Doubleday, New York, 1997

Allende, Isabel. *Paula*
HarperCollins, New York, 1996

Browne, Sylvia with Lindsay Harrison. *The Other Side and Back: A Psychic's Guide to Our World and Beyond*
Dutton, New York, 2000

Byock, Ira, M.D. *Dying Well: Peace and Possibilities at the End of Life*
Free Press, A Division of Simon & Schuster, Inc, New York, 2002

Byock, Ira, M.D. *The Four Things That Matter Most: A Book about Living.*
Free Press, A Division of Simon & Schuster, Inc., New York 2004

Callanan, Maggie and Kelley, Patricia. *Final Gifts:*

Understanding the Special Awareness, Needs, and Communications of the Dying.
Poseidon Press, New York, 1992

Dowling Singh, Kathleen. *The Grace in Dying: How We Are Transformed Spiritually as We Die.*
Harper SanFrancisco, New York, 2000

Eadie, Bette. *Embraced by the Light*
Gold Leaf Press, Placerville CA, 1992

Fry, Virginia Lynn. *Part of Me Died, Too.*
Dutton Children's Books, New York 1995

Grollman, Earl A. *Straight Talk about Death for Teenagers.*
Beacon Press, Boston, 1993

Grollman, Earl A. *Talking about Death: A Dialogue Between Parent and Child.*
Beacon Press, Boston, 1990

Groopman, Jerome, M.D. *The Measure of Our Days: New Beginnings at Life's End.*
Penguin, United States, 1998

Kubler-Ross, Elisabeth, M.D. *On Death and Dying.*
MacMillan Publishing Co., Inc. New York 1969

Levine, Steven. *Healing into Life and Death.*
Anchor Books reissue edition, New York, 1989

Moody, Raymond W.M.D. *Life after Life.*

Harper SanFrancisco, New York, 2001 (2nd edition)

Oliver, Mary. *New and Selected Poems.*
Beacon Press, Boston, 1992

Rodegast, Pat and Stanton, Judith. *Emmanuel Book II: The Choice for Love*
Bantam Dell Publishing, New York 1989

Saunders, Dame Cecily. OM DBE FRCP Video tape: *The Evolution of Hospice Care.*
St. Christopher's Hospice, London 2000

Soygal Rinpoche. *The Tibetan Book and Living and Dying*
HarperSanFransico, New York 1998

Tobin, Daniel R., M.D., with Kitty Lindsey. *Peaceful Dying*
Perseus Books, Reading MA. 1999

Van Praagh, James. *Talking to Heaven: A Medium's Message of Life after Death*
New York, Dutton, Nov 1997

Wheeler, Karla. *Afterglow: Signs of Continued* Love
Quality of Life Publishing Co 2002

Printed in the United States
90342LV00002B/109/A

9 781413 779981